WHAT YOU MUST KNOW ABOUT
STROKES
HOW TO RECOVER FROM A STROKE
AND PREVENT ANOTHER STROKE

AMYTIS TOWFIGHI, MD
LAURA J. STEVENS, MSCI

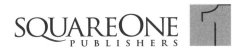

SQUAREONE
PUBLISHERS

COVER DESIGNER: Jeannie Rosado
IN-HOUSE EDITOR: Michael Weatherhead
TYPESETTER: Gary A. Rosenberg

Square One Publishers
115 Herricks Road
Garden City Park, NY 11040
(516) 535-2010 • (877) 900-BOOK
www.squareonepublishers.com

Library of Congress Cataloging-in-Publication Data
Names: Towfighi, Amytis, author. | Stevens, Laura J., 1945– author.
Title: What you must know about strokes : how to recover from a stroke and
    prevent another stroke / Amytis Towfighi, MD and Laura J. Stevens, MSci.
Description: Garden City Park : Square One Publishers, [2020] | Includes
    bibliographical references and index. |
Identifiers: LCCN 2019048816 (print) | LCCN 2019048817 (ebook) | ISBN
    9780757004834 (paperback) | ISBN 9780757054839 (ebook)
Subjects: LCSH: Cerebrovascular disease—Treatment. | Cerebrovascular
    disease—Prevention. | Brain—Diseases.
Classification: LCC RC388.5 .T625 2020 (print) | LCC RC388.5 (ebook) | DDC
    616.8/1—dc23
LC record available at https://lccn.loc.gov/2019048816
LC ebook record available at https://lccn.loc.gov/2019048817

Printed in the United States of America

10   9   8   7   6   5   4   3   2   1

Contents

Part IV. Life after a Stroke

$\mathcal{A}$cknowledgments

I would like to thank my coauthor, Laura J. Stevens, MSci, for being an absolute joy to work with, and Rudy Shur and Michael Weatherhead at Square One Publishers for their support. Thank you, Sabrina Rubin, my dear friend, for providing input from the perspective of a writer and sister of a young stroke survivor. I would like to thank my colleagues Valerie Hill, PhD, OTR/L, and Wendy Burton, MA, CCC-SLP, who gave insightful comments on the therapy sections. I would also like to thank my parents (Manijeh and Parviz Towfighi), brothers (Ali and Arya Towfighi), and fiancé, Sean McBride, who have always been there for me. Finally, I owe a debt of gratitude to my patients and their families for sharing their most vulnerable moments with me and inspiring me with their incredible courage and perseverance.

Amy Towfighi, MD

I would like to thank my coauthor, Amy Towfighi, MD, for agreeing to work on this book with me, and Rudy Shur and Michael Weatherhead at Square One Publishers, who allowed this book to see the light of day. I would also like to thank Dr. Pradeep, Dr. Galland, and James Sparandeo for helping me move forward after my stroke. Besides aiding me in my rehabilitation, Dr. Pradeep also inspired me to write this book. Special thanks go to my physical therapists, Sarah and Cathy, and my occupational therapists, Adam and Johanna. They helped me regain my balance and coordination, and prepared me to drive, live safely, and play tennis again. They also contributed greatly to my knowledge of strokes and rehabilitation, and even read parts of this book's manuscript. Thanks also go to Joe Braden, my tennis teacher, who turned out to be very knowledgeable about coordination and balance, and who corresponded with my therapists about my progress and what to work on. He cheered me on every step of the way. Finally, big hugs of appreciation go to my dear sons, Jack and Jeff, for all their love, assistance, and encouragement. Thank you one and all!

Laura J. Stevens, MSci

Preface

My story began on July 12, 2017. I had gotten up and fed my cat and myself, and was relaxing in front of the TV to watch the morning news, which was extra troubling that day. Suddenly, I realized I couldn't move my left leg. I knew I was having a stroke. I felt utter terror, but I managed to press my Medic Alert button, which I had worn around my neck since acquiring it, thank God. Immediately, I heard a voice in the kitchen saying, "Are you all right, Mrs. Stevens?" I replied, "No I'm having a stroke. Please send help!"

It seemed like it took an eternity for the EMS to arrive. I tried to stand up and unlock the door. Stupid idea! I fell on my left side, injuring my ribs, which hurt for weeks. EMTs were able to enter the house because Medic Alert had given them the code to my lockbox containing my house key—like the one a realtor puts on your front door. They quickly assessed me and agreed I had likely experienced a stroke. They immediately alerted the hospital to assemble the stroke team. They also inserted an IV and asked me all kinds of questions.

The stroke team was waiting for me at the hospital—approximately ten nurses, doctors, and technicians. A neurologist would arrive a few minutes after I got there. Then I was off for a CAT scan to determine whether my stroke had been caused by a blood clot or a bleed. This was critical information, and it was found that I had experienced a blood clot, not a bleed. One modern medical miracle is a drug called TPA, which dissolves blood clots. It is helpful only if given shortly after a stroke, though, and if given to a patient with a bleed it could cause fatal bleeding. However, because my stroke had been caused by a blood clot and the CT scan had not shown any bleeding, they gave me TPA. The paralysis of my left side and face began to improve considerably and I entertained the naïve thought that perhaps I could go home that afternoon.

Of course, I didn't go home that afternoon. I spent two days in intensive care. The paralysis would come and go, and with it extreme restless leg syndrome. I couldn't keep my left leg from shaking violently, and soon both legs were jerking. Finally, they gave me medication to stop the shaking. I was out of bed the first day and was able to stand with help.

After two days, they took me by ambulance to a rehabilitation unit at a different hospital. My rehab doctor was great, and he and his team of therapists were pros. By then we knew I was going to be okay. I asked the doctor why I had had the stroke, as I didn't have any of the risk factors—I was thin, I exercised, my blood pressure was low, I did not have diabetes, I had never smoked, and my diet was stellar—lots of fruits and veggies, lots of whole grains, and very little red meat. He had no clear answer, but he emphasized that my lifestyle had clearly made the stroke less severe and would make my recovery faster and easier.

I was in the rehab hospital for about ten days. I had two immediate goals that spurred me on. The first was to play tennis again; the second was to go to Michigan in two weeks—a vacation my sons and I had been planning and looking forward to for months. In fact, my sons stood over my bed and said so sternly, "Now, Mom, you need to work *really hard* in rehab." They didn't mention the Michigan trip, but I could tell it was a large factor in their insistence that I work hard to recover—it was a large factor in my desire to recover quickly, too! They also notified all my friends and gave them specific times they could visit me so that I wouldn't become overtired.

I worked really hard. I slurred my speech for the first few days and was seen a couple of times by a speech therapist, who tested my speech and my ability to swallow. But I needed occupational and physical therapy sessions twice a day. I had the greatest therapists. They knew my goal was to go to Michigan soon. My PT would say, "Michigan," when the length of my steps was too short. He also knew my goal was to play tennis again, so a friend brought in my tennis racket and we hit balloons.

Yes, we went to Michigan on time. I had wanted to play a little tennis, but my sons nixed that—"No, Mom, your balance is not good enough," and they were right. We went for lots of short walks, and they said, "Michigan," whenever my steps were too short. I really wanted to shuffle, so I had to fight against that inclination. We gradually increased the distance. We had a great time, but I was sleepy and exhausted. I would almost fall asleep at breakfast. I had to take many naps over the course of a day, and I still slept well at night.

When we returned home, I attended months of OT and PT. My physical therapist said I wasn't ready for tennis, but we could work on that goal. I grabbed my racket and hit a tennis ball against a wall with my therapist holding on to me as support. I even tried to serve. We worked endlessly on my walking to make it normal. In OT we worked extensively on the skills needed for driving, especially trying to lower my reaction time. Eventually, my therapists told my doctor I was okay to drive if I could pass a driving test with a special therapist. I passed—another milestone crossed.

Finally, my PT said I was ready to try a little tennis. Fortunately, I had been taking lessons previous to my stroke, so I went back to the same instructor. He couldn't have been better—he was especially interested in balance and coordination. Some days he would say, "No backhand or serving today—your balance isn't good enough." And after each lesson, he would write a summary for my PT, spelling out what I needed to work on. It was months before I could get my serve over the net. I continue the tennis lessons today, and they have greatly improved my balance, movement, and coordination.

After leaving physical therapy, I had several periods when my balance and coordination were off, so I returned to PT and worked hard on those skills again. I still do balance exercises every day. Most of the time I am fine, but there are times when I'm wobbly—especially first thing in the morning and when I'm tired.

The idea to write this book was suggested to me by my rehab doctor soon after he learned I was a health book author. When I felt ready, I reached out for a coauthor. I was fortunate enough to connect with Amy Towfighi, MD—a renowned stroke expert. She said her passion was stroke research and better patient recoveries. I knew I had found the right person. Now that our book is finished, I feel the same sense of accomplishment I felt as I stepped back onto the tennis court—the sense of accomplishment that comes in reaching a once daunting goal.

Strokes usher in an unexpected period of change. I hope this book makes the changes that accompany a stroke a little easier to manage and the difficulties of recovery a little easier to overcome.

Just one more thing: In order to avoid awkward phrasing within sentences, the publisher has chosen to alternate between the use of male and female pronouns. Therefore, male pronouns are used when referring to stroke survivors or at-risk individuals, while female pronouns are used when referring to doctors or other members of the healthcare community.

Introduction

A stroke changes the lives of many people: the stroke survivor, his family members, and his friends. The first goal of this book is to help you understand what a stroke is. The second goal is to explain why strokes occur and how to reduce or eliminate their risk factors. The third goal is to help stroke patients recover from their strokes as much as possible. The final goal is to support caregivers, whether they are spouses, siblings, grown children, or dear friends.

Written by stroke specialist Amy Towfighi, MD, and health writer and stroke survivor Laura J. Stevens, MSci, *What You Must Know About Strokes* explains what happens during a stroke, how a stroke is treated in the hospital, the various aspects of the rehabilitation process, the difficulties stroke patients may encounter in returning home and how to address them, and how to prevent a second stroke.

Part I defines the event, describes the different types of strokes, and details the many effects they can cause. It also talks about the critically important warning signs of a stroke, which can help you save a stranger's life, a loved one's, or your own. It also discusses neuroplasticity—the amazing ability of the brain to form new networks to meet new needs, essentially "rewiring" itself, which is especially helpful after a stroke. Part I goes on to discuss the risk factors for stroke—high blood pressure, smoking, type 2 diabetes, poor diet, alcohol consumption, inactivity, and obesity. In fact, high blood pressure accounts for over half of all strokes. It is critical to understand these risk factors so you can help yourself or your loved ones decrease these risks and prevent a second stroke or avoid a first one altogether.

Part II explains what happens after a stroke patient reaches the hospital, how stressful this experience can be for both the patient and his loved ones, and how vital it is to get excellent care. By the time you read this book, this hospital period will likely be behind you or your loved one, but we are presenting this material to make the book complete for all readers. Part II discusses inpatient and out-patient rehabilitation—what to expect in therapy, the different forms of therapy, and the types of therapists and their training. Depending upon a stroke survivor's needs, he may receive occupational, physical, speech, vision, or other therapies. Part II also touches upon complementary therapies that have not been studied as much as standard therapies but about which you may have questions—for example, massage, music therapy, and acupuncture. It describes each therapy, details any research behind it, and gives our pertinent recommendations.

Part III is meant to help stroke survivors avoid having another stroke. Many patients who experience a first stroke will have another stroke if they don't work on their risk factors. Part III can help stroke survivors greatly reduce their risks of having a second stroke. For example, for a stroke patient who has high blood pressure—a critical risk factor for many stroke survivors—this part discusses ways in which he may bring it down, including medication, dietary changes, and exercise. In fact, because diet is critical in reducing stroke risk, we have devoted four chapters to this topic. Chapter 10 talks about protective nutrients, including certain vitamins, minerals, essential fatty acids, and antioxidants that will heal and protect the brain and blood vessels. Chapter 11 concentrates on foods and food components to limit or avoid completely, such as red meat, processed meat, saturated fat, trans fat, sodium, alcohol, sugar, and artificial sweeteners.

Chapter 12 discusses recommended foods that can help prevent strokes, such as whole grains, fruit, vegetables, lean protein (less beef protein, more chicken, fish, or plant protein), nuts, dairy and alternatives, and so on. It is not easy for a person to change his diet, but this book makes it easier, recommending healthy, delicious foods that will lead to better health. Chapter 13 offers menus for tasty daily meals and snacks, giving you an example of one week of menus and snack suggestions. It also explains how to choose healthy foods when dining out, and discusses assisted living and how to achieve a heart-and brain-healthy diet in this environment.

Part IV deals with stroke effects you cannot see, such as fatigue, depression, anxiety, pain, and sleep problems. Many stroke survivors have these problems, but there are ways to improve mood and lift depression, and this part of the book can show you how. In addition, it offers lots of practical advice about safety, addressing a stroke survivor's need for a safety-proofed home that has been organized so that it functions well for his new needs. It also talks about a stroke survivor's need to maintain a routine that includes getting all his meds on time, preparing healthy meals and snacks, going to outpatient rehab, and keeping appointments with his healthcare provider after he leaves the hospital.

Stroke patients have the ability to make improvements in recovery and avoid another stroke by going to all therapy sessions, doing appropriate exercises at home, choosing a healthy diet, taking appropriate medications, and seeing their doctors for all scheduled appointments. Rome wasn't built in a day, but this book can help stroke survivors lead better, healthier, and happier lives.

PART I

Learning about Strokes

1

What Is a Stroke?

U nless you or a loved one has experienced a stroke, this medical possibility may never have entered your mind. Yet strokes are the leading cause of disability and second leading cause of death worldwide. On average, every forty seconds, someone in the United States has a stroke. If you or someone you know has experienced one, it helps to understand what has taken place. It is also essential to know that anyone who has had a stroke is at increased risk of having another. In fact, 25 percent of all strokes occur in people who have already had strokes. Despite these alarming statistics, the good news is that, in addition to being able to predict and prevent strokes, we now have effective ways to treat stroke patients. Moreover, the brain has an incredible capacity to repair itself, and repeat strokes can be prevented.

This chapter discusses how and why specific types of strokes occur. It looks at symptoms that may appear during a stroke, making one easier to spot. The decisions made during the first minutes after a stroke are crucial to outcomes, so this chapter includes information on what should be done during this time period. Finally, it discusses prognosis after the event.

STROKES EXPLAINED

To better understand strokes, you need to first learn about blood and how the brain receives oxygen. Blood vessels that carry oxygen-rich blood to the body are called *arteries*. They divide into smaller blood vessels called *capillaries*, which connect to the *veins*. Oxygen in the bloodstream is delivered to the body's cells at the capillary level. Once this has been accomplished, veins carry oxygen-depleted blood back to the heart. This blood circulates through the lungs, picks up more oxygen, and returns to the heart, which then pumps this oxygen rich-blood through arteries to the organs. The main artery originating from the heart is called the *aorta*. The aorta branches into smaller arteries which supply brain cells, also known as *neurons*.

Advice for Caregivers
WHY UNDERSTANDING STROKE-RELATED WORDS IS IMPORTANT

Becoming acquainted with the medical terms and explanations found in this chapter will help you better understand what happens during a stroke, communicate with the healthcare team, and relay beneficial information to a loved one who has had a stroke. Don't hesitate to ask questions if things are unclear. The healthcare team knows this situation is likely overwhelming and will be happy to explain and reiterate information.

Almost half of blood (55 percent) consists of *plasma,* which is a yellow liquid that carries nutrients such as glucose, proteins, fatty acids, and so on. The remaining percentage is made up of three kinds of blood cells. *Red blood cells* give blood its color and are responsible for carrying oxygen to all cells. *White blood cells* help the body fight infections. Finally, *platelets* help prevent excessive bleeding after an injury.

As we age, *plaque,* which is made up of fat, cholesterol, calcium, and other substances found in the blood, begins to accumulate in our arteries. This process starts when we are teenagers and is impacted by blood pressure, cholesterol, diabetes, diet, smoking, and genetics. It can lead to narrowing and hardening of arteries.

Plaques are also prone to rupturing. When they do, platelets and clotting proteins in plasma rush to the site of injury to repair it, forming a *blood clot.* A blood clot—also referred to as a *thrombus*—is a thick clump of blood that forms after an injury and "plugs" the hole at the injured site. Blood clots can occur in both veins and arteries, but strokes, except in rare circumstances, are related to clots in arteries. A clot can completely block a blood vessel (causing an *occlusion*), or a piece of it may break off (this piece is called an *embolus*) and travel down the path of a blood vessel, eventually blocking a smaller blood vessel. (See Figure 1.1 below.) This blockage is known as an *embolism*. This process is similar to what happens during a heart attack. If a plaque ruptures in an artery of the heart, a blockage may result that deprives the heart of oxygen, causing a *heart attack*. If it ruptures in an artery leading to the brain, a blockage may occur that deprives the brain of oxygen, causing what is known as an *ischemic stroke*.

In addition to plaque build-up in arteries leading to strokes, the walls of arteries can become fragile when they have been exposed to high blood pressure, type 2 diabetes, smoking, cholesterol, or stimulant drugs (such as cocaine or amphetamines). Once they have become fragile, they can burst, causing bleeding in the brain, also known as a *hemorrhagic stroke*.

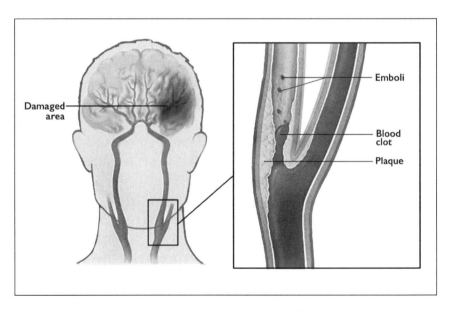

Figure 1.1. Blood Clots and Brain Damage

The majority of strokes (85 percent) are of the ischemic variety, and it is important to understand the difference between each type, as their symptoms and treatments may differ. For example, a severe headache that comes on suddenly is more commonly a warning sign of a hemorrhagic stroke. In both cases of stroke, depending on the location of the injured cells in the brain, certain parts of the body may no longer function as they should.

Ischemic Strokes

Ischemic strokes are typically subdivided by the underlying cause: plaque in large arteries (*large artery atherosclerosis*), small vessel disease, clots that originate in the heart (*cardioembolic stroke*), or "other" types.

Large artery atherosclerosis means there is plaque build-up in the walls of arteries leading to the brain. When plaque accumulates on the walls of arteries, causing hardening and narrowing, it can reduce the flow of oxygen-rich blood to the brain. Alternatively, a plaque can rupture, causing a clot to form, which can then either block an artery or break off and travel to a smaller artery in the brain, obstructing blood flow. Conditions that lead to plaque build-up include high blood pressure, poor diet, smoking, physical inactivity, abnormal cholesterol levels, and type 2 diabetes.

Small vessel disease refers to narrowing of the small arteries that originate from the larger arteries leading to the brain. The major factors responsible for small vessel disease are high blood pressure and type 2 diabetes, although cholesterol and smoking also likely play a role. These small arteries can become blocked, causing an ischemic stroke.

A stroke caused by a clot originating in the heart, known as a cardioembolic stroke, can be caused by numerous conditions, including a mechanical heart valve, heart attack, heart failure, clot in the heart, infection of a heart valve, or an irregular heart rhythm known as *atrial fibrillation.*

Strokes in the "other" category include strokes due to a tear called a *dissection* in the arteries leading to the brain, blood-clotting disorders (as can be seen in individuals with rheumatic diseases such as lupus), sickle cell disease, or stimulant medications or drugs (including cocaine, methamphetamines, and over-the-counter pharmaceuticals such as pseudoephedrine).

Sometimes, the cause of a stroke cannot be determined. In these cases, more diagnostic tests will likely need to be done to find out why it occurred. Even with extensive testing, the cause may not be apparent in approximately 20 percent of cases.

Hemorrhagic Strokes

Hemorrhagic strokes are divided into those that bleed into the brain, which are known as *intracerebral hemorrhages,* and those that bleed into the space between the brain and the skull, which are called *subarachnoid hemorrhages.* An intracerebral hemorrhage is usually caused by high blood pressure or by a protein known as *amyloid,* which builds up in the small arteries of the brain as we age. Other causes include blood-thinning medications, structural abnormalities of arteries or veins, stimulant drugs, and excessive alcohol use.

A subarachnoid hemorrhage is typically caused by the rupture of an outpouching, or balloon-like bulge, of the wall of an artery, otherwise known as an *aneurysm.* It can also result from abnormalities of arteries or veins.

Transient Ischemic Attack (TIA)

A *transient ischemic attack,* or TIA, occurs when the supply of blood to an area of the brain is blocked but then restored. As its name implies, a TIA is temporary, and damage to the brain is not sustained. Even though the symptoms of a TIA subside, it is critical to go to the hospital after experiencing one to determine why it happened and to start medications to prevent a future stroke. In some cases, an urgent intervention such as surgery may be indicated. The short-term risk of having a stroke after a TIA is as high as 10 percent at two days, and 17 percent at ninety days.

WHAT CAUSES STROKES?

While some strokes are not preventable, the overwhelming majority of strokes can be prevented by changes to lifestyle habits and control of key risk factors. In fact, five modifiable risk factors account for over

80 percent of all strokes: high blood pressure, smoking, abdominal obesity, poor diet, and physical inactivity. High blood pressure is by far the most important cause of stroke, accounting for half of all cases. Other common causes of stroke include an irregular heart rhythm (atrial fibrillation), a dissection (tear) in an artery leading to the brain, and blood-clotting disorders. Chapter 2 on page 17 discusses the risk factors for stroke in detail.

STROKE EFFECTS

The overall effects of a stroke depend on the area of the brain that has been affected. Different parts of the brain are associated with different functions. When a particular area of the brain is deprived of oxygen or injured by bleeding during a stroke, the symptoms that manifest will be related to the bodily functions associated with this area.

There are numerous "stroke syndromes"—constellations of symptoms that correlate to the part of the brain affected by a stroke. In general, each side of the brain controls the other side of the body. Therefore, if a person has a stroke that affects the *right motor cortex*, he may suffer paralysis of the left side of his body. If a person has a stroke that affects the *left sensory cortex*, he will experience numbness on the right side of his body. A stroke in the *right occipital lobe* affects vision in the left visual field, whereas a stroke in *left occipital lobe* affects vision in the right visual field.

The location of language in the brain depends on whether an individual is left-handed or right-handed. In individuals who are right-handed, language is processed predominantly in the left side of the brain. For about 50 percent of left-handed people, however, language is processed predominantly in the right side of the brain. Therefore, a stroke in the left side of the brain would not affect language skills in these left-handed individuals. Although a left-handed person may exhibit slightly differently symptoms than a right-handed person would in relation to the exact same stroke, the collection of possible stroke symptoms remains the same. In light of this fact, it is important to learn these signs and know what to do when they appear.

The old real estate adage "location, location, location" also applies to strokes. A tiny (one centimeter in size) stroke in the frontal cortex may cause minimal symptoms, whereas a stroke of comparable size in the brainstem, where numerous pathways converge, can cause complete paralysis of one side of the body, numbness on one side of the body, or double vision. In short, the part of the brain affected by a stroke determines the resultant symptoms.

Arteries and Stroke Symptoms

Since different arteries supply blood to specific parts of the brain, some knowledge of these blood vessels can help you understand the aftermath of a stroke.

The brain receives its blood supply from two sources: the *internal carotid arteries*, which are paired arteries (i.e., one artery is found on each side of the brain) located at the front, or anterior, of the brain; and the vertebral arteries, which are located at the back, or posterior, of the brain.

Each internal carotid artery branches into a *middle cerebral artery* and an *anterior cerebral artery*. The vertebral arteries located on the right and left side of the neck join to form the *basilar artery*, a single artery that feeds the *brainstem*. The brainstem allows signals to travel between the brain and the spinal cord. The basilar artery then splits into *two posterior cerebral arteries*.

The anterior and posterior arteries join to create an important formation of arteries known as the *Circle of Willis* at the base of the brain. The Circle of Willis is helpful because it enables other arteries to feed the brain if one artery is blocked.

Stroke syndromes can be defined by the arteries that supply blood to the brain. A *left middle cerebral artery stroke* can cause weakness in the right side of the face, right arm, and right leg; numbness of the right side of the face, right arm, and right leg; difficulty speaking and understanding; difficulty looking to the right; inability to see the right visual field; and slurred speech. A *right middle cerebral artery stroke* can cause weakness in the left side of the face, left arm, and left leg; numbness of the left side of the face, left arm, and left leg; difficulty looking to the left; inability to see the left visual field; neglect (lack of attention to) the left; and slurred speech. (See Table 1.1 on page 13.)

A *posterior cerebral artery stroke* can result in an inability to see the visual field of the opposite side of the affected side of the brain and difficulty with memory. (In other words, a left posterior cerebral artery stroke will cause blurring of the right field of vision, and vice versa.) An *anterior cerebral artery stroke* can cause weakness in one leg (depending on the side of the brain affected), problems in controlling urination, and personality changes.

A blood clot in the vertebral or basilar artery can lead to a range of symptoms that include dizziness, problems with balance, falls, weakness or numbness on one side of the body, double vision, and hiccups.

TABLE 1.1. STROKE LOCATION AND ITS ASSOCIATED EFFECTS

Affected Artery	Most Common Symptoms
Left middle cerebral artery stroke	• Weakness in the right side of face, right arm, and right leg • Numbness of the right side of face, right arm, and right leg • Difficulty speaking and understanding (in right-handed individuals and 50 percent of left-handed individuals) • Difficulty looking to the right • Inability to see the right visual field • Slurred speech
Right middle cerebral artery stroke	• Weakness in the left side of face, left arm, and left leg • Numbness of the left side of face, left arm, and left leg • Difficulty looking to the left • Inability to see the left visual field • Neglect (lack of attention to) the left • Slurred speech
Posterior cerebral artery stroke	• Inability to see the visual field of the opposite side of the affected side of the brain • Poor memory
Anterior cerebral artery stroke	• Weakness in one leg (depending on the affected side of the brain) • Urinary incontinence • Personality changes

COMMON WARNING SIGNS

You may save your life, a loved one's life, or the life of a stranger by knowing the warning signs of a stroke. Over the years, stroke treatment options have improved dramatically. We now have treatments that are highly effective if given within hours of symptom onset. We also have medications to reduce the risk of a second stroke and therapies to enhance recovery. The key to taking advantage of stroke treatments is calling 911 at the first sign of a stroke.

Using the acronym BE FAST can help you recall the main stroke warning signs and remember what to do if you or someone near you begins to experience any of them.

B: Balance

E: Eyes

F: Facial droop

A: Arm weakness

S: Speech slurred or difficulty speaking

T: Time to call 911

If you think someone is having a stroke, check his balance. Is he having difficulty standing or walking? Is he having any difficulty seeing? Is he experiencing double vision or an inability to see on one side? Ask him to smile. Does one side of his face droop? Ask him to raise both arms. Does one arm drift down? Ask him to repeat a phrase. Is his speech slurred or difficult to understand? Does he have difficulty understanding you? If you spot any of these signs, call 911 immediately.

STROKE CENTERS

If you witness someone having a stroke and immediately call 911, emergency medical personnel will transport him to the nearest hospital capable of managing strokes, and often will notify the hospital prior to arrival, so that the entire stroke team will be ready. On the way to the hospital, emergency medical technicians, or EMTs, will measure his vital signs and insert an IV into one of his veins so he can receive drugs at the hospital immediately. Therefore, if you see someone experiencing stroke warning symptoms, call 911 for immediate care, and don't try to drive the patient to the hospital yourself. Precious time will be lost in assembling the stroke team, and he won't get the treatment he needs in a timely fashion. Remember: Every second counts during a stroke.

WHY CALL 911?

Dr. Jeffrey Saver, one of the most influential stroke neurologists, in a landmark paper, quantified just how much brain is lost during every second of a stroke. He estimated that in a typical large vessel stroke, 120 million neurons (nerve cells), 830 billion synapses (connections between nerve cells), and 714 km (447 miles) of myelinated fibers (cell parts that work like electrical wires transmitting signals) are lost each hour. In each minute, 1.9 million neurons, 14 billion synapses, and 12 km (7.5 miles) of myelinated fibers are destroyed. In fact, a brain deprived of oxygen ages 3.6 years each hour without treatment. These staggering figures underlie why it's important to seek treatment as soon as possible and halt the damage.

A nationwide independent organization known as the Joint Commission currently awards certificates of distinction to hospitals equipped to manage strokes and ensure better outcomes related to stroke care. In many cities throughout the United States, ambulance routing protocols ensure that individuals with stroke symptoms are routed to hospitals with the ability to manage strokes. *Primary stroke centers* have demonstrated that they are able to deliver timely, appropriate care and meet key quality metrics related to treating strokes with clot-busting medications when necessary, taking measures to avoid complications, and starting appropriate medications to prevent additional strokes. *Comprehensive stroke centers* and *thrombectomy-capable centers* have even more specialized services, such as managing an aneurysm or pulling a clot out of an artery.

PROGNOSIS FOR RECOVERY

During the first few days after a stroke, the medical team will provide treatments to minimize damage to the brain and supportive care to ensure that the brain is getting adequate blood flow and oxygen. It will also take measures to minimize complications that may result from the stroke. Once a stroke survivor is beyond those first few days, the prognosis for recovery is promising, given the brain's remarkable ability to create new networks. The brain has a property called *neuroplasticity*, meaning it can form new networks throughout life. When existing networks are damaged by a stroke, new ones can form. This ability of the brain to compensate for injury underlies much of the recovery after stroke. In later chapters, you will learn how therapy can be used to take advantage of the brain's innate neuroplasticity.

CONCLUSION

A stroke is a common condition that has a tremendous impact on people's lives, yet it is treatable and preventable, and the brain has a remarkable ability to repair itself once it has experienced a stroke. The majority of strokes (85 percent) are ischemic strokes, the type caused by a blockage of an artery leading to the brain. The remaining 15 percent of strokes involve bleeding into or around the brain. Strokes express themselves in different ways, depending on which part of the brain has been affected.

Most strokes can be prevented by changes to lifestyle habits and control of key risk factors. Five factors in particular are responsible for four out of five strokes: high blood pressure, smoking, abdominal obesity, poor diet, and physical inactivity. Among these factors, high blood pressure is by far the most important cause of stroke, accounting for half of all cases. The next chapter discusses the aforementioned risk factors and others in greater detail.

Finally, don't forget these two words: BE FAST. They stand for balance, eyes, face, arm, speech, and time to call 911. The better you are able to recognize the warning signs of a stroke, the quicker you will be able to get help, and this speed can make all the difference in terms of outcome. When it comes to strokes, the sooner a stroke patient reaches appropriate care, the better the result. Remember: Time is brain.

2

Who Is at Risk?

It is crucial to know the factors that put you at risk of having a stroke, particularly if you have already had a stroke and wish to avoid experiencing another one. This information can also help you spot stroke risk factors in others and show those at-risk how to mitigate or eliminate these factors. As you read this chapter, you will come to understand how simple it is to recognize these risk factors. While some of these factors cannot be easily altered, the vast majority of them can be changed.

Understanding whether a person is at risk of having a TIA, a first stroke, or recurrent strokes is aided by looking at the available science and statistics. This chapter not only names stroke risk elements but also explains why they may present a danger to your health in more ways than one.

STROKE STATISTICS

Each year, approximately 800,000 individuals in the United States experience a stroke. Three-quarters of these strokes are first attacks. The remainder represents repeat events in individuals who have previously had a stroke or TIA. Age, race, ethnicity, and sex affect stroke risk. Stroke risk increases with age. Nevertheless, strokes can occur in younger people, too—approximately 30 percent of stroke survivors are under the age of 65. Under the age of eighty, men are more likely to have a stroke than women, but in later years, women have an equal or higher risk of stroke than men. In addition, since women live longer than men, and the risk of stroke is higher in the elderly, more women than men are living with the effects of having had a stroke. With respect to race and ethnicity, black and Hispanic individuals are more likely than whites to experience a stroke, while Asians and Native Americans have fewer strokes than white people. A strong family history of stroke also puts a person at risk of having a stroke.

THE STROKE RISKOMETER

If you want a quick and easy way to determine your risk of stroke, there's an app for that. Endorsed by the World Stroke Organization, the Stroke Riskometer is a free app for smartphones and tablets that can inform you of your risk of having a stroke in the next five or ten years. It also shows you how your risk level compares with the risk level of someone of the same age but who has no risk factors. The website https://www.strokeriskometer.com provides more information.

SEVEN MODIFIABLE RISK FACTORS

Although strokes can be caused by a multitude of factors, there are seven key modifiable risk factors responsible for the overwhelming majority of cases:

1. High blood pressure
2. Smoking
3. Type 2 diabetes
4. Abnormal cholesterol
5. Obesity
6. Lack of physical activity
7. Poor diet

In fact, high blood pressure, smoking, abdominal obesity, physical inactivity, and poor diet account for 82 percent of ischemic and 90 percent of hemorrhagic strokes in the world. Many other factors increase stroke risk, including an abnormal heart rhythm known as atrial fibrillation, depression, mechanical heart valves, heavy alcohol use, illicit drug use (such as cocaine and methamphetamine), sleep apnea, migraines, contraceptive use, and pregnancy.

TABLE 2.1. LIFE'S SIMPLE 7S CALCULATOR

Risk Factor	Poor (0)	Intermediate (1)	Ideal (2)	Score
Blood Pressure (mmHg) **SBP: Systolic Blood Pressure** **DBP: Diastolic Blood Pressure**	SBP ≥ 140 or DBP ≥ 90	SBP = 120–139 or DBP = 80–89 or treated to less than 120/80	< 120/80 without a hypertension drug	
Smoking	Current smoker	Former smoker or quit less than one year ago	Never smoker or quit more than one year ago	
Fasting Glucose (mg/dL)	≥ 126	100–125 or treated to less than 100	< 100	
Total Cholesterol (mg/dL)	≥ 240	200–239	< 200	
Body Mass Index (kg/m²)	≥ 30	25–29.9	18.5–25	
Physical Activity	None	1–149 minutes a week of moderate activity or 1–74 minutes a week of vigorous activity	At least 150 minutes a week of moderate activity or 75 minutes a week of vigorous activity	
Diet	0–1	2–3	4–5	
	One point for each of the following daily components: • Fruits and vegetables, about 4.5 cups a day • Fish, 3.5 ounces about two times a week • Sodium, less than 1,500 mg a day • Sweets or sugar-sweetened beverages, less than 450 kcal a week • Whole grains, about 3 servings a day			
Total Score				

In light of the seven key factors listed above, the American Heart Association has developed a set of goals for ideal cardiovascular health. Entitled "Life's Simple 7s," it addresses each of these seven factors and states that ideal cardiovascular health (and thus a reduction in stroke risk) may be accomplished by quitting smoking, engaging in regular physical activity, eating a healthy diet, and maintaining normal weight, blood pressure, cholesterol, and blood sugar levels. (Information on how to change these factors and minimize the risk of having another stroke appears in Chapter 9 on page 126.) Remember that "Life's Simple 7s" can be controlled.

A person should know where he stands with each of Life's Simple 7s, particularly if he is a stroke survivor. Table 2.1 (see page 19) is designed to help people calculate their cardiovascular risks according to the American Heart Association's set of categories. A score for each risk factor should be marked (from 0 to 2), and then the seven scores should be added together to find their sum. A score of 0–4 corresponds to poor cardiovascular health; a score of 5–9 corresponds to intermediate cardiovascular health; and a score of 10–14 corresponds to optimal cardiovascular health.

For those who have already had a stroke, Table 2.2 (below) can act as go-to guide to goals for these risk factors.

TABLE 2.2. GOALS AFTER A STROKE

Risk Factor	Goal
Blood Pressure	Less than 130/80 mmHg
Smoking	Do not smoke
Blood Sugar	Hemoglobin A1c less than 7%
Cholesterol	LDL cholesterol level less than 70 mg/dL
Weight	BMI 18.5–24.9 kg/m²
Physical Activity	At least three sessions of 20–60 minutes of moderate intensity aerobic activity a week
Diet	Consume recommended servings of fruit and vegetables, whole grains, low-fat dairy, fish, nuts or legumes, and healthy vegetable oil (avoid salt, sugar, saturated or trans fat)

■ HIGH BLOOD PRESSURE

High blood pressure, also known as *hypertension,* is by far the strongest risk factor for stroke. In fact, nearly half of all strokes are due to this condition. High blood pressure can lead to stroke in two different ways. First, high blood pressure contributes to fatty plaque build-up in the large arteries supplying oxygen to the brain. As described in Chapter 1, when a plaque ruptures, clotting factors rush to the site of injury to repair it. This causes a fresh clot to occur at the site of the plaque. The clot can obstruct the blood vessel, or pieces of the clot can travel up to the brain, depriving the brain of oxygen, resulting in an ischemic stroke. In addition, over time, high blood pressure weakens the smaller blood vessels inside the brain, making them prone to burst. When these tiny blood vessels burst, bleeding into the brain, or intracerebral hemorrhage, occurs.

Fortunately, lowering blood pressure reduces stroke risk. In fact, in someone who has had a stroke or TIA, lowering blood pressure reduces the likelihood of having another stroke by 24 percent and heart attack by 21 percent. For a person who has had a stroke, the goal blood pressure will likely be less than 130/80 mmHg. In rare cases, someone with a prior stroke requires a slightly higher goal, so stroke patients should make sure to ask their healthcare providers what their goals should be. The following table (Table 2.3) is a reference guide to blood pressure categories. Tips to lower high blood pressure may be found in Chapter 9.

TABLE 2.3. BLOOD PRESSURE CATEGORIES

Category	Systolic Pressure, mmHg (first number)		Diastolic Pressure, mmHg (second number)
Normal	Less than 120	and	Less than 80
Elevated	120-129	and	Less than 80
Stage 1 hypertension	130-139	or	80-89
Stage 2 hypertension	140 or higher	or	90 or higher
Hypertensive Crisis	Higher than 180	and/or	Higher than 120

Measuring Blood Pressure

There are several key elements involved in blood pressure control. First, blood pressure should be monitored at home. A blood pressure monitor may be purchased at a local pharmacy. Cuffs that are placed on the upper arm are more accurate than wrist cuffs. People with blood pressure monitors should get into the habit of checking blood pressure twice a day. Keep in mind that blood pressure normally varies throughout the day, and can be affected by stress and physical activity. It should be checked only after the person being tested has been sitting calmly for five minutes. Individuals should not speak or move while checking blood pressure.

Blood pressure measurements should be recorded in a blood pressure log, notebook, or app. People who are concerned with their blood pressure levels should ask their healthcare providers what their levels should be and, if testing at home, at what level should these healthcare providers be notified. Recorded measurements should be taken to appointments and shared with healthcare providers. These logs will help doctors adjust blood pressure medications if necessary. Any person who is not taking his blood pressure medication as prescribed should tell his doctor. She should also be made aware of the reason for his not taking this medication as prescribed, whether the reason is unwanted side effects, forgetfulness, or any other reason. A doctor will work with a patient to find a regimen that makes sense for him.

White Coat Hypertension

For some people, blood pressure levels increase during check-ups in a healthcare provider's office. If a patient's blood pressure reading is elevated in his doctor's office but returns to normal levels outside a healthcare setting, this elevated reading is considered *white coat hypertension*. This is another reason to check blood pressure at home.

■ SMOKING

Smoking increases the risk of having a stroke by almost twofold and contributes to 15 percent of all ischemic strokes. Smoking is a major cause of plaque build-up in arteries. In addition, smoking makes blood prone to forming clots. Smoking can affect cholesterol levels, causing triglyceride levels to rise and lowering the "good" cholesterol, known as high-density lipoprotein, or HDL. Finally, smoking can make it harder to control blood sugar levels. Fortunately, after quitting smoking, stroke risk declines to a non-smoker's risk in approximately two to five years. There are numerous aids to quit smoking, which are discussed in Chapter 9.

Secondhand smoke also increases stroke risk and worsens outcomes after stroke, so it is important to avoid secondhand smoke if possible. At-risk individuals should not to allow anyone to smoke in their houses or cars. If there are smokers in their circles of friends, they should be encouraged to quit—for the health of those around them and their own health.

■ TYPE 2 DIABETES

Type 2 diabetes is associated with a twofold to twelvefold increase in stroke risk. It accounts for 7.5 percent of ischemic strokes worldwide. In the United States, approximately one third of stroke survivors have diabetes. While type 1 diabetes is an autommimune disease that almost always begins in childhood and is likely related to genetics, type 2 diabetes, which accounts for 95 percent of all diabetic cases, is typically acquired later in life and may be avoided or improved with lifestyle choices. As a result, type 2 is the form discussed in this book.

Blood sugar levels are tightly regulated by the body. Carbohydrates are broken down into sugars in the bloodstream. The body releases insulin to break down these sugars. Over time, in people who have persistently high blood sugar levels, the body becomes resistant to insulin, insulin levels become chronically elevated, and blood sugar levels remain high. When blood sugar levels remain high, diabetes develops. *Hemoglobin A1c* is a blood test that determines a person's average blood sugar level over the past three months. A normal hemoglobin A1c level is less than 5.7 percent. Those who have levels between 5.7 percent and 6.5 percent have a precursor to type 2 diabetes called *prediabetes*. Those whose hemoglobin A1c is over 6.5 percent have diabetes. The following table (Table 2.4) shows normal, prediabetic, and diabetic levels of fasting blood sugar and hemoglobin A1c.

TABLE 2.4. BLOOD SUGAR MEASUREMENTS

Blood tests	Normal	Prediabetic	Diabetic
Fasting blood glucose	Less than 120 mg/dL	120 to 125 mg/dL	126 mg/dL or higher
Hemoglobin A1c	Less than 5.7%	5.7 to 6.5%	More than 6.5%

Common symptoms of type 2 diabetes include thirst, frequent urination (often at night), unintentional weight loss, hunger, blurry vision, numbness, tingling or burning pain in the feet, fatigue, dry skin, sores that heal slowly, and frequent infection. Sometimes this condition has no symptoms at all, so it is important to get a blood test regardless of whether or not symptoms occur. Individuals who are overweight, over forty-five years old, not physically active, or have a parent, brother, or sister with type 2 diabetes are at a higher risk of aquiring this condition. Other people who are at a higher risk include those who are black, Hispanic, or Native American, and those who have had diabetes during pregnancy.

Type 2 diabetes has numerous detrimental effects on the body. It contributes to plaque development in the walls of arteries, increasing a person's risk of stroke, heart attack, kidney disease, and eye disease. It also damages nerves, causing burning pain and numbness. People with type 2 diabetes who develop damage to the nerves, called *neuropathy,* often don't feel if they have injured their feet. They develop foot ulcers that are slow to heal, and may need amputations if the wounds don't heal. The good news is that type 2 diabetes can be controlled with diet and medication.

For those who have prediabetes, it is important to alter diet, quit smoking, and embark on a physical activity regimen to reduce the likelihood of developing type 2 diabetes. If someone has type 2 diabetes, in addition to becoming physically active and eating a healthier diet, it is essential for him to control his blood glucose, blood pressure, and cholesterol. Blood sugar levels should be checked before each meal and at bedtime. A person can develop an understanding of how the food he eats affects his blood sugar levels. A reasonable target for hemoglobin A1c is less than 7 percent. A safe blood pressure goal for a diabetic is less than 130/80 mmHg.

Chapter 9 provides information on how to reduce fasting blood sugar and hemoglobin A1c by changing diet, taking medications, and exercising.

■ ABNORMAL CHOLESTEROL

Cholesterol is a waxy, fat-like substance found in the body. The body makes all the cholesterol it needs, but cholesterol is also found in foods from animal sources, such as meat, egg yolks, and cheese. If there is too much cholesterol in the blood, it can contribute to plaque formation, which can build up in blood vessels, increasing a person's risk of experiencing a stroke or heart attack.

There are several types of cholesterol: *low-density lipoprotein* (LDL) cholesterol, *high-density lipoprotein* (HDL) cholesterol, and *triglycerides*, another type of fat. LDL is called the "bad" cholesterol because a high LDL level leads to a build-up of plaque in arteries. HDL is called the "good" cholesterol because it carries cholesterol from other parts of the body back to the liver, which then removes this cholesterol from the body. When you eat, your body converts any calories it doesn't need to use right away into triglycerides. Triglycerides are stored in fat cells. Later, hormones release triglycerides for energy between meals. If an individual regularly eats more calories than he burns, particularly from high-carbohydrate foods, he may have high triglycerides, also known as *hypertriglyceridemia*. High levels of LDL and triglycerides and low levels of HDL cholesterol each result in a higher stroke risk. Table 2.5 (see page 27) describes the ideal levels of HDL cholesterol, LDL cholesterol, total cholesterol, and triglycerides.

A variety of factors can cause abnormal cholesterol levels, including age, genetics, diet, weight, and physical inactivity. Cholesterol tends to rise with age, and high cholesterol can run in families. In addition, race plays a role, with black people typically having higher LDL levels than white people.

Diet, weight, and physical activity levels can be controlled. Eating food that is high in saturated fat can raise LDL cholesterol and triglycerides levels. A diet rich in sugar and refined carbohydrates leads to lower HDL levels, higher triglyceride levels, and higher LDL levels.

Belly fat (abdominal obesity) and a sedentary lifestyle can result in low HDL and high triglyceride levels. In addition, type 2 diabetes lowers the HDL cholesterol levels and increases LDL cholesterol levels.

High cholesterol typically has no symptoms, so it is important to get a blood test. Physical activity, diet, and certain medications can improve abnormal cholesterol levels.

■ OBESITY

Being overweight or obese is associated with a higher risk of having a stroke. Obesity is determined according to height and weight. The *body mass index,* or BMI, is a measure of a person's relative size based on weight and height. It's calculated by dividing weight in kilograms by height in meters squared, but if you would rather not do the math to figure out you own BMI, you can consult Table 2.6 on pages 28 and 29, or use an online BMI calculator.

If you already know your BMI, Table 2.7 (see page 30) can show you where you stand in terms of weight category.

Those who are *overweight* are 1.4 times more likely to have a stroke than those who are not. Those who are *obese* are nearly twice as likely to have a stroke. Approximately 22 percent of ischemic strokes (one in five) and 25 percent (one in four) of hemorrhagic strokes are due to obesity.

If you are overweight or obese *and* your extra weight is around your waist rather than your hips, then you have *abdominal obesity.* Abdominal obesity, in particular, is associated with several problems, including high blood pressure, low levels of HDL, high levels of triglycerides, and insulin resistance. This constellation of factors is called *metabolic syndrome.* Individuals with metabolic syndrome are more prone to having a stroke.

■ POOR DIET

Diets that are rich in saturated fat, salt, sugar, and refined carbohydrates increase stroke risk, whereas diets rich in fruits and vegetables, whole grains, monounsaturated fat, and fish lower it. Unfortunately, eating a typical American diet is a major risk factor for stroke. This

TABLE 2.5. IDEAL CHOLESTEROL AND TRIGLYCERIDES

Type of cholesterol	Ideal Level (mg/dL)
Total Cholesterol	Less than 200
LDL Cholesterol	Less than 70
HDL Cholesterol	Men: over 40 Women: over 50
Triglycerides	Less than 150

general eating pattern is full of harmful food components with few nutrients. It raises blood pressure and blood glucose, causes weight gain, raises LDL cholesterol while decreasing HDL cholesterol, and increases the risks of stroke and heart disease. Because diet is so important, four chapters in this book are dedicated to adopting a healthy diet. (See Chapters 10, 11, 12, and 13.)

■ ALCOHOL USE

While light to moderate alcohol use (less than one drink per day for women and two drinks per day for men) may help protect you from a stroke, it's a slippery slope. Heavy drinking increases the risk of stroke nearly twofold. In fact, heavy drinking is responsible for 5 percent of ischemic and 10 percent of hemorrhagic strokes worldwide.

Alcohol increases stroke risk through numerous mechanisms. Drinking too much alcohol raises blood pressure, the number one risk factor for stroke. Drinking can also change the way the body responds to insulin, increasing the risk of type 2 diabetes. Alcoholic drinks tend to be high in calories, so drinking regularly can make it more difficult to maintain a healthy weight. Drinking excessive amounts of alcohol can trigger an abnormal heart rhythm (atrial fibrillation), which increases stroke risk by five times. Finally, alcohol use can lead to liver damage. People with liver disease are at higher risk of bleeding, including bleeding in the brain.

If you are a drinker, the American Heart Association recommends limiting your alcohol to one serving of alcohol per day for women,

TABLE 2.6. BODY MASS INDEX TABLE

	Normal						Overweight					Obese					
BMI	19	20	21	22	23	24	25	26	27	28	29	30	31	32	33	34	35
Height (inches)									Body Weight (pounds)								
58	91	96	100	105	110	115	119	124	129	134	138	143	148	153	158	162	167
59	94	99	104	109	114	119	124	128	133	138	143	148	153	158	163	168	173
60	97	102	107	112	118	123	128	133	138	143	148	153	158	163	168	174	179
61	100	106	111	116	122	127	132	137	143	148	153	158	164	169	174	180	185
62	104	109	115	120	126	131	136	142	147	153	158	164	169	175	180	186	191
63	107	113	118	124	130	135	141	146	152	158	163	169	175	180	186	191	197
64	110	116	122	128	134	140	145	151	157	163	169	174	180	186	192	197	204
65	114	120	126	132	138	144	150	156	162	168	174	180	186	192	198	204	210
66	118	124	130	136	142	148	155	161	167	173	179	186	192	198	204	210	216
67	121	127	134	140	146	153	159	166	172	178	185	191	198	204	211	217	223
68	125	131	138	144	151	158	164	171	177	184	190	197	203	210	216	223	230
69	128	135	142	149	155	162	169	176	182	189	196	203	209	216	223	230	236
70	132	139	146	153	160	167	174	181	188	195	202	209	216	222	229	236	243
71	136	143	150	157	165	172	179	186	193	200	208	215	222	229	236	243	250
72	140	147	154	162	169	177	184	191	199	206	213	221	228	235	242	250	258
73	144	151	159	166	174	182	189	197	204	212	219	227	235	242	250	257	265
74	148	155	163	171	179	186	194	202	210	218	225	233	241	249	256	264	272
75	152	160	168	176	184	192	200	208	216	224	232	240	248	256	264	272	279
76	156	164	172	180	189	197	205	213	221	230	238	246	254	263	271	279	287

				Extreme Obesity														
36	37	38	39	40	41	42	43	44	45	46	47	48	49	50	51	52	53	54

Body Weight (pounds)

172	177	181	186	191	196	201	205	210	215	220	224	229	234	239	244	248	253	258
178	183	188	193	198	203	208	212	217	222	227	232	237	242	247	252	257	262	267
184	189	194	199	204	209	215	220	225	230	235	240	245	250	255	261	266	271	276
190	195	201	206	211	217	222	227	232	238	243	248	254	259	264	269	275	280	285
196	202	207	213	218	224	229	235	240	246	251	256	262	267	273	278	284	289	295
203	208	214	220	225	231	237	242	248	254	259	265	270	278	282	287	293	299	304
209	215	221	227	232	238	244	250	256	262	267	273	279	285	291	296	302	308	314
216	222	228	234	240	246	252	258	264	270	276	282	288	294	300	306	312	318	324
223	229	235	241	247	253	260	266	272	278	284	291	297	303	309	315	322	328	334
230	236	242	249	255	261	268	274	280	287	293	299	306	312	319	325	331	338	344
236	243	249	256	262	269	276	282	289	295	302	308	315	322	328	335	341	348	354
243	250	257	263	270	277	284	291	297	304	311	318	324	331	338	345	351	358	365
250	257	264	271	278	285	292	299	306	313	320	327	334	341	348	355	362	369	376
257	265	272	279	286	293	301	308	315	322	329	338	343	351	358	365	372	379	386
265	272	279	287	294	302	309	316	324	331	338	346	353	361	368	375	383	390	397
272	280	288	295	302	310	318	325	333	340	348	355	363	371	378	386	393	401	408
280	287	295	303	311	319	326	334	342	350	358	365	373	381	389	396	404	412	420
287	295	303	311	319	327	335	343	351	359	367	375	383	391	399	407	415	423	431
295	304	312	320	328	336	344	353	361	369	377	385	394	402	410	418	426	435	443

TABLE 2.7. WHERE YOU STAND USING BMI

BMI Ranges (kg/m²)	Category
From 18.5 to 24.9	Normal
From 25 to 29.9	Overweight
30 and above	Obese

and two for men. If you are a non-drinker, it recommends not starting. The following table (Table 2.8) shows the definitions of a "drink" according to the type of alcohol.

TABLE 2.8. STANDARD SERVINGS OF DIFFERENT TYPES OF ALCOHOL

Alcoholic Beverage	Size of Standard Drink	Alcohol Content in Grams and Percentage
Beer	12 fluid ounces	14 grams, or 5%
Wine	5 fluid ounces	14 grams, or 12%
Distilled spirits (80 proof)	1.5 fluid ounces	14 grams, or 40%

■ LACK OF PHYSICAL ACTIVITY

Among the seven key vascular risk factors, physical inactivity is responsible for approximately one-third of all strokes. As you likely already know, physical activity can have numerous positive health effects, including lowering body weight and blood pressure, and improving cholesterol levels.

The American Heart Association guideline recommendations for preventing a first stroke are to exercise at a moderate or vigorous intensity for at least thirty minutes a day, at least five times a week. Moderate exercise intensity feels somewhat hard. Your breathing quickens but you are not out of breath; you develop a light sweat after about ten minutes of activity; and you can carry on a conversation but can't sing. Vigorous intensity feels hard. Your breathing is deep and rapid; you develop a sweat after only a few minutes; and you can't say more than a few words without pausing for a breath. The intensity depends on your fitness level. For someone who has had a stroke or TIA, regular physical activity will reduce the risk of another stroke or a heart attack. Of course, if a stroke has affected a person's coordination and muscle strength, his healthcare provider and physical therapist will help him develop an exercise plan.

■ DEPRESSION

You may be surprised to learn that depression is a risk factor for stroke. Depression is a common medical illness that negatively affects how you feel, think, and act. It is normal to feel sad or depressed at times, but when intense sadness lasts for weeks and interferes with your life, it may be due to clinical depression. Depression is likely caused by a combination of genetic, biological, environmental, and psychological factors, and is often accompanied by changes in chemicals in the brain, including serotonin and norepinephrine. It can be triggered by major life changes, trauma, or stress, and is commonly associated with certain medical conditions.

Depression can cause a variety of symptoms, including sadness, loss of interest or pleasure in activities you once enjoyed, changes in appetite, trouble sleeping or sleeping too much, loss of energy, slowed movements and speech, feelings of worthlessness or guilt, difficulty concentrating or making decisions, and thoughts of death or suicide. Symptoms must last at least two weeks to classify as depression. Depression, for reasons that are unclear, is a risk factor for stroke. In addition, depression is a common symptom after stroke, affecting approximately one-third of stroke survivors. (Chapter 14 on page 234 discusses depression after stroke.)

Are You Depressed?

The following questionnaire (Table 2.9) is a good tool for detecting depression. Based on the answers circled, a person must calculate the total of each column and then add these totals together to get his overall score. A score of 0 to 4 suggests minimal or no depressive symptoms. Scores of 5 to 9 indicate mild symptoms that should be reviewed by a healthcare provider. Scores of 10 to 14 indicate moderate depression, which means treatment options, including counseling or medication, should be discussed with a doctor. A score of 15 or above suggests at least moderately severe depression, which means the help of a healthcare provider is needed as soon as possible.

TABLE 2.9. PATIENT HEALTH QUESTIONNAIRE 9 (PHQ-9) DEPRESSION QUESTIONNAIRE

(Circle the number to indicate your answer.)

Over the last two weeks, how often have you experienced any of the following problems?	Not at all	Several days	More than half the days	Nearly every day
Little interest or pleasure in doing things	0	1	2	3
Feeling down, depressed, or hopeless	0	1	2	3
Trouble falling asleep or staying asleep, or sleeping too much	0	1	2	3
Feeling tired or having little energy	0	1	2	3
Poor appetite or overeating	0	1	2	3
Feeling bad about yourself—or that you are a failure or have let yourself or your family down	0	1	2	3
Trouble concentrating on things, such as reading the newspaper or watching television	0	1	2	3
Moving or speaking so slowly that other people have noticed? Or the opposite—being so fidgety or restless that you are moving around a lot more than usual	0	1	2	3
Thoughts of being better off dead or of self-harm	0	1	2	3
Column Total	0	+___	+___	+___
Overall Total	=			

■ DISSECTION (TEAR)

A stroke can be caused by a tear in an artery, also known as a dissection. This event can be caused by trauma from a car accident, fall, or contact sport, or rapid head movements, which can be seen in chiropractic manipulation or trauma. Certain people are more prone to dissections due to genetic weakness in blood vessels. Typically, dissection is treated with either a blood-thinning agent, such as warfarin, or an antiplatelet medication, such as aspirin or clopidogrel. Those who have had a dissection should talk to their healthcare professionals about what medications to take, and any restrictions in physical activity that may apply.

■ HORMONAL BIRTH CONTROL

Hormonal birth control can increase the risk of stroke, particularly in smokers. Several mechanisms may be responsible for this increase in stroke risk, including increasing blood pressure and making the blood more prone to forming clots. Stroke risk increases with estrogen dose. Hormonal contraceptives that do not contain estrogen, such as the progestin-only *intrauterine device*, likely do not increase risk of stroke.

For healthy young women with no vascular risk factors, the risk of having a stroke associated with hormonal contraceptives is small. In women with other risk factors, however, such as older age, high blood pressure, cigarette smoking, or migraine headaches (particularly migraines with sensory or visual aura, such as flashing lights), hormonal contraceptives should be discouraged. The FDA recommends against the use of oral contraceptives in women over thirty-five who smoke. Women who have had a stroke should talk to their healthcare providers before starting hormonal birth control.

■ PREGNANCY

Pregnancy increases the risk of a stroke. During pregnancy and the four weeks after delivery, a woman's stroke risk increases more than twofold. There are numerous changes in the body during pregnancy that increase the likelihood of a pregnant woman having a stroke, including clotting factors in the blood, changes in blood vessels, and dehydration. In addition, there are numerous possible complications of pregnancy that increase the risk of stroke, including preeclampsia (high blood pressure accompanied by damage to the kidney, liver, or lung) and gestational diabetes (diabetes that develops during pregnancy). The time period around delivery is the highest risk time for a pregnant woman. In order to prevent stroke during pregnancy, low-dose aspirin from the twelfth week of gestation until delivery may be recommended for women with high blood pressure or previous pregnancy-related high blood pressure.

■ DRUG USE

Numerous drugs, both legal and illegal, can lead to strokes. Stimulants such as cocaine, methamphetamines, and MDMA (ecstasy) can cause strokes by several mechanisms. First, they can cause sudden severe narrowing or spasm of the arteries to the brain, reducing blood supply to the brain. Second, they can cause a sudden, dramatic increase in blood pressure, leading to bleeding in the brain. Third, they can cause long-term damage to the arteries of the brain, resulting in strokes even years after drug use.

Intravenous drug use can cause an infection of the bloodstream, which can infect the heart valves. When heart valves are infected, clumps of bacteria and cells that have formed at the site of infection can break off and travel to the arteries of the brain, causing strokes. Opioids such as heroin or prescription opioids (e.g., hydrocodone, oxycodone, codeine, morphine, fentanyl) can lower blood pressure, breathing, and oxygen delivery to the brain.

In addition to illicit drugs, there are a number of readily available products that have been associated with stroke, including energy drinks, weight loss supplements, and over-the-counter cold medications (typically those that contain pseudoephedrine).

■ HEART-RELATED STROKE RISKS

Approximately one out of four ischemic strokes originates in the heart. The heart pumps blood to the brain, so there are numerous ways in which it can be responsible for a stroke. First, clots can form in the chambers of the heart (either the left atrium or left ventricle) due to an abnormal heart rhythm, heart attack, or weakened heart that does not pump effectively. In addition, clots, infection, or scar tissue can develop on the valves of the heart and travel to the brain.

Finally, one out of four people have a connection between the left and the right side of the heart, known as a *patent foramen ovale,* or PFO. In people with a PFO, a clot formed in a deep vein in the body (typically a vein in a leg), also known as *deep vein thrombosis,* or DVT, can travel through the heart and go to the brain, causing a stroke. Risk factors for DVT include prolonged periods of immobility (such as lying in a hospital bed or sitting on a plane), dehydration, and trauma.

Atrial Fibrillation

Atrial fibrillation is a disorder of the heart rhythm that results in an irregular heartbeat. When the heart beats irregularly, the blood in the left atrium of the heart (one of the four chambers of the heart) is stagnant, making it prone to forming clots. A clot can travel to the brain, causing a stroke. Risk factors for atrial fibrillation include advanced age (it's more common in older individuals), high blood pressure, underlying heart disease (such as history of heart attack), binge drinking (having more than five drinks in two hours for men, and more than four drinks in two hours for women), family history, sleep apnea, and thyroid problems.

Heart Failure

Heart failure does not mean that the heart is not working. It means that the heart works less efficiently than normal. As a result, blood moves through the heart and body at a slower rate, and the heart cannot pump enough oxygen and nutrients to meet the body's needs. The chambers (typically the two ventricles) of the heart either stretch or become stiff and thickened. When the heart doesn't pump efficiently, the blood in the heart can become prone to forming clots, which can be delivered to the brain, causing a stroke.

Heart failure has several causes. The most common causes are high blood pressure and heart attack. Other causes include damaged heart valves, infection or inflammation of the heart muscle, excessive use of alcohol, type 2 diabetes, obesity, and high cholesterol levels.

Heart failure can cause numerous symptoms, including fatigue, weight gain, shortness of breath, increased urination at night, low energy, and swelling of the leg, ankle, or foot. A person with heart failure should ask his healthcare professionals what he can do to reduce his risk of having a stroke.

Endocarditis

Endocarditis is inflammation of the heart valves. When it is caused by an infection in the bloodstream, it is called *infective endocarditis*. When heart valves are infected, clumps of the infection and cells can break off and travel to the brain, causing a stroke. People with underlying heart conditions such as rheumatic heart disease or heart valve replacement or repair are most prone to this condition. Typically, infective endocarditis occurs when the bloodstream is infected with bacteria. Symptoms include fevers, chills, fatigue, aching joints and muscles, night sweats, unexplained weight loss, and swelling in the legs, feet, or abdomen. Diagnosing endocarditis usually involves an ultrasound of the heart and blood tests. Endocarditis is treated with antibiotics. In severe cases, heart valve replacement may be needed if the valve has become damaged and the heart is not pumping effectively.

Endocarditis can also be caused by rheumatologic conditions such as *systemic lupus erythematosus*. In rheumatologic conditions, scar tissue can develop on the valve and break free, traveling to the brain and causing a stroke.

Mechanical Heart Valve

When heart valve disease has progressed to the point at which medicine does not provide relief from symptoms, a clinician may recommend surgery to repair the heart valve. There are two broad categories of heart valve replacements: mechanical and bioprosthetic. Mechanical valves have the advantage that they are durable and last many years. The downside is that clots can develop on them. If a blood clot develops on the valve and dislodges, it can enter the circulation to the brain, causing a stroke. For this reason, people with mechanical valves are typically prescribed blood thinners. Bioprosthetic valves are made of pig, cow, or horse tissue. These are not as prone to clotting, so people with bioprosthetic valves typically don't need long term blood thinners.

Paradoxical Embolism

A *paradoxical embolism* occurs when a clot in the veins of the legs or pelvis travels through the heart or lungs to the brain. The only way this event can occur is if you have a shunt (a small hole or passage) in the arteries of the lungs or between the left and right side of the heart. Shunts in the lungs are rare; shunts in the heart, however, are more common. The most common type of heart shunt is the previously mentioned patent foramen ovale, or PFO, which approximately one out of four people have. PFOs typically do not cause any symptoms, but if you develop a clot in your legs and have a PFO, the clot has a passageway to reach the brain.

A PFO can be diagnosed by injecting a salt-water solution that contains tiny air bubbles into the veins and using an ultrasound to watch the heart or arteries in the head. If a shunt is present, bubbles will be seen passing from the right to the left side of the heart. There have been a number of trials to determine whether to close PFOs in stroke survivors whose strokes are believed to have been the result of a PFO. They have shown that PFO closure lowers stroke risk in certain stroke survivors. Stroke patients should ask their healthcare providers if their strokes were related to a PFO. If a stroke is associated with a PFO, a healthcare provider can recommend whether the PFO needs to be closed. As mentioned, risk factors for clots in the legs include prolonged immobility (such as experienced during air travel or a stay in the hospital), trauma, and dehydration.

COVID-19 AND STROKES

Although the most common symptoms of the illness known as COVID-19 are cough and fever, this infection can also cause more serious symptoms that require hospitalization, including pressure in the chest and breathing difficulty. Clinicians have also noticed, however, an alarming association between some hospitalized COVID-19 patients and strokes, even in young adults, who would not normally be at risk. While scientists are not certain this new disease can cause strokes, they have speculated that the virus may bind to cells inside blood vessels, triggering an immune system reaction, which can lead to clotting. These blood clots may then travel to the brain and result in strokes.

CONCLUSION

Those who know the risk factors for a TIA, first stroke, and recurrent strokes can take actions to reduce or eliminate them. For example, smokers can try to quit. A person who has high blood pressure can try to reduce it. Blood pressure goals should be discussed with a professional, who can recommended ways to achieve blood pressure readings that won't promote a stroke. Likewise, people can find out how to improve their cholesterol scores, lower their fasting blood sugar and Hemoglobin A1c numbers, drop some weight, and come up with a realistic exercise plan that they will enjoy and maintain. Behavioral change is hard, but there are tools and tips to help achieve these goals. (See Part III on page 125.)

The next chapter discusses what happens in the hospital after a stroke. A stroke patient may be alarmed by all the doctors, nurses, and other clinicians rushing around and doing lots of different things to assess his condition. But he can rest assured that they are experienced and know exactly how to diagnose the cause of a stroke, give him the proper treatment, minimize complications, and initiate therapy to aid in recovery.

PART II

Experiencing a Stroke

3

*W*hat to Expect in the Hospital

Since strokes happen unexpectedly, common reactions are shock, panic, fear, and anxiety. For most stroke patients and their loved ones, the first days immediately following a stroke are a blur full of unfamiliar people—doctors, nurses, technicians, and hospital staff—asking questions, performing tests, and explaining diagnoses and treatment options in technical language. Some treatments require consent forms, and it can be very difficult for a stroke patient to make an informed decision at such a time.

Although everyone may look like they are in a hurry and things may even seem a little chaotic, it is important to know that the professionals involved in the situation have been well trained to make a stroke patient comfortable, save his life, and prevent as much stroke-related damage to his brain as possible. This chapter describes what happens in the hospital during the first twenty-four hours after a stroke, which are critical to recovery, and then it discusses what happens in the hospital after that first day, when recovery begins.

THE FIRST TWENTY-FOUR HOURS

In the first twenty-four hours after a stroke, a stroke patient's healthcare team will perform three key functions: *supportive care*, *diagnosis*, and *treatment*. This section discusses each of these functions in series, but it is worth noting that they may occur simultaneously.

Supportive Care

In any medical emergency, healthcare providers will first address the ABCs: airway, breathing, and circulation. The airway refers to the passage from the nose and mouth to the lungs. In the event of a stroke, a patient may become very sleepy and unable to keep his airway open or breathe on his own. If this happens, it may be necessary for his healthcare provider to place a tube down his throat via his mouth and attach it to a breathing machine, or ventilator.

The need for a ventilator varies from patient to patient. It is related to the location and severity of a stroke, and the presence of other medical conditions. A ventilator can be a life-saving tool, and it is typically used only temporarily. In most cases, a patient can be weaned off a ventilator and the tube removed. If a patient needs a ventilator for more than two weeks, a procedure may be recommended wherein the tube is inserted through a hole in his neck, making the patient more comfortable in the long run and allowing him to speak. Often, a patient will not need to be on a breathing machine but may require supplemental oxygen. This oxygen is usually delivered by a medical device called a *nasal cannula.* This device consists of a small plastic tube that splits into two prongs, which are placed in the nostrils.

Circulation is the next key component of supportive care. Most of the time, a stroke patient will have high blood pressure when he arrives at the hospital. If his stroke is a result of bleeding into or around the brain (hemorrhagic), then the emergency team will lower his blood pressure with medication, which is often given through an intravenous line. If his stroke is ischemic (a blockage of one of the arteries), then high blood pressure will actually help deliver blood and oxygen to the areas of the brain at risk of damage. As a result, high blood pressure will likely be tolerated in the first couple of days after a stroke—unless clot-busting medication was used as an emergency measure.

Reducing the risk of aspiration is another key factor in supportive care. *Aspiration* occurs when liquid or food travels down the wrong pipe and enters the lungs rather than the stomach. Stroke patients often have difficulty swallowing, a condition called *dysphagia.* Symptoms of dysphagia include problems when starting to swallow; choking;

coughing or gagging while swallowing; liquid coming out of the nose after trying to swallow; weak voice; drooling; poor tongue control; and loss of the gag reflex. Dysphagia increases the risk of aspiration. In addition, when food or liquid enters the lungs, a lung infection known as *pneumonia* may result.

Two key interventions help prevent aspiration. First, the head of a patient's bed should elevated to an angle of 30 degrees. If the head of the bed is flat, then the risk of aspiration increases. If a patient is sitting up straight, delivery of blood to the brain may be compromised. Therefore, an angle of 30 degrees is the sweet spot to ensure blood gets to the brain and the risk of aspiration is reduced. Second, a stroke patient should not drink or eat anything (even pills with water) before a bedside swallow evaluation has been performed. A bedside swallow exam may be done by a nurse, physician, physician assistant, nurse practitioner, or speech therapist. Most bedside swallow exams start with a brief cognitive screen; continue with an examination of the movement of the lips, tongue, and face; and end with a swallow test of three ounces of water.

During a stroke patient's brief cognitive screen, a healthcare provider will ask him questions such as, "What is your name?", "Where are you right now?", and "What year is it?" During the second part of the evaluation, she will check if he can close his lips, move his tongue, and smile symmetrically. Finally, she will ask him to drink three ounces (90 ml) of water from a cup or with a straw in several swallows. She will check for signs of coughing or choking during or after drinking. If there is no difficulty swallowing, then she will likely determine that it is safe for him to take pills by mouth with water. Often, a speech therapist will do a more thorough swallow evaluation in order to determine if eating is safe.

Control of blood sugar is another key to supportive care. Both high blood sugar and low blood sugar have been shown to worsen the outcome of a stroke. Blood sugar frequently spikes in the event of a stroke as a result of the stress it places on the body. Insulin given an injection under the skin, or *subcutaneously,* may be necessary to bring blood sugar back down to a normal level.

If a stroke patient has a fever, the source should be identified and treated, and medication such as acetaminophen (Tylenol) will likely be used to lower the temperature. Studies have found that low tempera-ture and high temperature are both associated with worse outcomes; therefore, maintaining a normal body temperature is important.

Diagnosis

A patient's medical team will administer a brief neurologic exam to determine the severity of his stroke. The National Institutes of Health (NIH) Stroke Scale is a quick bedside clinical test performed by healthcare professionals. The NIH Stroke Scale includes evaluations of a patient's level of consciousness, eye movements, visual fields (the ability to see things to the left and right of midline), facial sym-metry, strength in arms and legs, ataxia (inability to move each limb smoothly), sensation, language, and speech. The severity of a stroke may impact treatment options.

A *computed tomography scan*, commonly known as a CT scan, of the head is one of the key diagnostic tests for a stroke. A CT scan takes less than five minutes to complete and provides several important bits of information. It can detect blood; therefore, it's the method of choice to differentiate between a stroke that involves bleeding (hem-orrhagic) and a stroke that involves a blocked blood vessel (ischemic). Each type of stroke is managed in a different way. For example, a medical team will manage a hemorrhagic stroke by lowering blood pressure and reversing any blood thinners that a patient may have taken. On the other hand, in the case of an ischemic stroke, a medical team will tolerate high blood pressure in a patient and often adminis-ter blood-thinning medications.

A healthcare provider may also do additional imaging of a patient's blood vessels with a *CT angiogram*, or CTA. In a CTA, con-trast dye is injected into a vein and scans are taken that show the contrast moving through the blood vessels. This test demonstrates whether there are any blockages of the arteries. During the contrast injection, *perfusion* studies may also be done. Perfusion refers to the passage of fluid through the circulatory system to an organ or tissue—in this case, blood flow to the brain—and perfusion studies can inform a patient's healthcare team of brain tissue that has been damaged due to lack of oxygen (ischemia), or of brain tissue that is experiencing a decrease in blood flow but hasn't died yet. The goal will be to save tissue at risk by administering medication to break up the clot, physically removing the clot with a device, or allowing blood pressure to remain a little higher than normal. A patient's treatment choice will depend on the time since onset of his stroke, the damage that has already been done by his stroke, the symptoms of his stroke, and his and his family's preferences.

Treatment of Ischemic Stroke

As described in Chapter 1, an ischemic stroke occurs when a blood clot blocks an artery leading to the brain, thus depriving it of oxygen. A blood clot is formed when platelets and clotting proteins in plasma combine to form a clump of cells. While blood clots can form in both arteries, which take oxygen-rich blood from the heart to other organs, and veins, which bring oxygen-depleted blood back to the heart, strokes are, except on rare occasions, connected to blood clots that have formed in arteries.

When a clot blocks an artery that supplies blood to the brain, it can cause an ischemic stroke. Clots typically form in arteries that have been hardened by *atherosclerosis*. Atherosclerosis is the medical term used to describe a condition in which hard plaques form in the arteries, causing the arteries to narrow over time. While this condition can affect anyone, it frequently occurs in connection with high blood pressure, high cholesterol, type 2 diabetes, and smoking.

Atherosclerotic plaque is covered by a fibrous cap that separates the soft interior contents from the bloodstream. If this cap becomes eroded (ulcerates) or breaks (ruptures), the contents (including tissue fragments, fat-filled cells, and cholesterol) are exposed and released into the bloodstream. These tissue fragments stimulate clot formation. A clot can narrow an artery or block the artery entirely, depriving part of the brain of the oxygen it needs to survive. Treatment of ischemic stroke includes attempts to: (1) dissolve the clot with *thrombolytic* (clot-busting) medication; (2) remove the clot via mechanical *thrombectomy* (using a mechanical device); and (3) prevent the clot from expanding by using *antiplatelet* or *anticoagulant* medication (together known as *antithrombotics*).

Dissolving the Clot

In the event of an ischemic stroke, a thrombolytic medication, which is a drug designed to break up blood clots, may be used. The medication used for an ischemic stroke is called *alteplase*. Alteplase is a laboratory-manufactured *tissue plasminogen activator,* or tPA. tPA is an enzyme that the body produces to help dissolve clots. When it is manufactured in a laboratory, it is called *recombinant tissue plasminogen activator,* or rtPA. Alteplase is an rtPA that has been shown to improve outcomes after stroke if it is given within four and half hours of symptom onset. A stroke patient's healthcare team will spend some time to determine his "last known well time," which refers to the last time the patient did not display any symptoms of a stroke. If a patient spoke with someone at 9 PM, went to bed at 10 PM, and awoke at 7 AM unable to speak or understand others, and is unable to give a history to his healthcare team, the last known well time would be 9 PM. His stroke could have occurred at any point between 9 PM and 7 AM, but there is no way of knowing exactly when it happened. Therefore, for purposes of determining whether or not rtPA can be given, the last known well time would be 9 PM.

Numerous trials have shown that alteplase, when administered within three hours of a patient's last known well time, is associated with improved outcomes. An additional study extended this window to four and half hours in select patients.

While mild, moderate, and severe strokes may be treated with alteplase in most patients, there are certain circumstances that preclude its use. These circumstances include a last known well time of over four and half hours, bleeding into or around the brain, large areas of damage to the brain, infection of heart valves, and a tear in the aorta. In other circumstances, treatment with alteplase has the potential to cause harm, including ischemic stroke in the previous three months, severe head trauma in the previous three months, brain or spinal surgery in the previous three months, gastrointestinal cancer or recent gastrointestinal bleeding (in the past three weeks), prior bleeding in the brain, bleeding issues or clotting abnormalities, and brain tumor. In any of these cases, a healthcare provider will need to consider and discuss with the patient or his loved one the pros and cons of treatment with alteplase.

Mechanical Removal of the Clot (Mechanical Thrombectomy)

If a patient has a blood clot in one of the major arteries leading to his brain and meets certain criteria, he may be a candidate for mechanical removal of the clot with an expandable wire-mesh tube called a *stent retriever*. This device can be used up to twenty-four hours since last known well time (but ideally within the first six hours) if certain criteria are met. If he is eligible for this procedure, his healthcare team will insert a catheter into his femoral artery through an incision in the groin area. The catheter is moved up the artery to the site of the blocked brain artery. When it reaches the clot, the stent retriever is deployed. The stent then expands, grabs on to the clot, and is threaded out of the body along with the clot. With removal of the clot, blood flow to the part of brain is restored.

Clinical trials for mechanical thrombectomy have demonstrated positive results in certain cases. In these cases, patients experienced speedier recoveries and improved chances of regaining independence when their clots were removed with stent retrievers as opposed to being treated with rtPA alone. If a patient is a candidate for both alteplase and thrombectomy, his team will do both. Mechanical clot retrieval is currently not performed instead of giving alteplase, although such trials are underway.

An ischemic stroke patient must meet certain criteria in order to be eligible to undergo a mechanical thrombectomy. It is typically used for moderate to severe strokes. The blood clot must be in the internal carotid artery or the first segment of the middle cerebral artery, although a healthcare provider may choose to perform a mechanical thrombectomy in a different location based on special circumstances. There must be no evidence of widespread damage visible on an imaging test, and treatment should generally be started within six hours of symptom onset.

Antiplatelet Medication

As mentioned earlier in this chapter, blood clots are typically made of platelets, red blood cells, and clotting proteins. In the event of atherosclerotic plaque rupture or injury to an arterial wall, these cells and clotting factors are recruited to the site of injury to form a clot. If the clot narrows or blocks the artery, blood flow slows down, causing the clot to get even bigger. There are two types of medications that are used to prevent clots from getting bigger: anticoagulants (which slow the time it takes for blood to clot) and antiplatelet medication (which prevents platelets from clumping together). Both are considered blood thinners, although neither one actually thins the blood. In most cases of ischemic stroke, antiplatelet medication is used.

The oldest and most commonly used antiplatelet medication is aspirin. Aspirin has been shown in many trials to reduce risk of a subsequent stroke and should be given within the first twenty-four hours of a stroke. There are a few instances when aspirin should not be given to a stroke patient: (1) if there is bleeding in the brain; (2) if alteplase has recently been administered (in which case, twenty-four hours must elapse before giving aspirin); and (3) if there is another condition increasing the risk of bleeding. Other than in these scenarios, aspirin therapy is standard. Other antiplatelet medications include clopidogrel (Plavix), extended-release dipyridamole and aspirin (Aggrenox), cilostazol (Pletal), and ticagrelor (Brilinta). In some cases, combination therapy with aspirin and clopidogrel or aspirin and cilostazol may be used initially.

Anticoagulants

Anticoagulants are a stronger type of blood thinner than antiplatelet medication. Examples of anticoagulants include warfarin, dalteparin, enoxaparin, fondaparinux, dabigatran, rivaroxaban, apixaban, and edoxaban. There are only a few instances in which anticoagulants are used, such as the presence of a clot in the heart, an irregular heart rhythm (atrial fibrillation), or a clot in a vein.

Maintaining Perfusion (Blood Flow) to the Brain

As specified earlier, it is critical to maintain perfusion, or blood flow, to the brain tissue at risk in order to prevent an ischemic stroke from expanding. In addition to giving clot-busting medication, mechanically removing the clot, and using antiplatelet medication, doctors can do various other things to maximize blood flow to the brain. First, they can keep the head of the bed at 30 degrees, unless there is a concern for raised pressure in the brain, in which case, they can raise the head of the bed. Second, they can give saline (salt water) through an intravenous catheter. Finally, they can let blood pressure autoregulate by avoiding medication to lower blood pressure. As explained earlier, blood pressure usually increases during a stroke. This reaction is a good protective mechanism to ensure blood flow to the brain. Doctors treat blood pressure only if the top number (systolic) goes above 220 mmHg in someone who has not received alteplase, and above 185 mmHg in someone who has received alteplase. The threshold is lower for those who have received alteplase because alteplase can cause bleeding. In some cases, doctors administer medications to increase blood pressure in order to maintain blood flow to the brain.

Treatment of Hemorrhagic Stroke

Approximately 15 percent of strokes are hemorrhagic, meaning they are caused by bleeding into or around the brain. As stated in Chapter 1, there are two types of hemorrhagic stroke: intracerebral hemorrhage and subarachnoid hemorrhage. An intracerebral hemorrhage is defined by bleeding into the brain tissue. It can be caused by high blood pressure, a condition called cerebral amyloid angiopathy, blood-thinning medication, alcohol use, malformations of blood vessels, or drug use. A subarachnoid hemorrhage is defined by bleeding around the brain. It is usually caused by a ruptured aneurysm or trauma. Other causes include drug use (typically stimulant drugs, such as cocaine), ruptured veins, and a tear in an artery leading to the brain.

The treatment of a hemorrhagic stroke will vary depending on whether it is an intracerebral or subarachnoid hemorrhage. Intracerebral hemorrhage is treated by lowering blood pressure, reversing any blood thinners, and occasionally surgically removing blood. In the event of a subarachnoid hemorrhage, the healthcare team will search for an aneurysm. If one is found, the doctor will secure it with surgery or an endovascular procedure (via the femoral artery in the groin) to prevent rebleeding. The blood in the subarachnoid space, on the surface of the brain, can irritate the other blood vessels coursing through this space and supplying the brain with blood. This irritation can trigger *vasospasm,* a condition in which arterial spasm results in constriction of the affected arteries. These narrowed arteries limit blood flow to the brain and could lead to an ischemic stroke.

Therefore, individuals with a subarachnoid hemorrhage are at risk of an ischemic stroke. To prevent this occurrence, doctors typically use a type of medication called a calcium channel blocker, which prevents the muscles of the arteries from contracting excessively, thus blocking vasospasm. In addition, patients with subarachnoid hemorrhage are typically monitored with serial ultrasounds of the arteries to the brain to look for signs of vasospasm.

AFTER THE FIRST TWENTY-FOUR HOURS

The first twenty-four hours are busy with supportive care, diagnostic tests, and treatment. After this period, supportive care, evaluation, and treatment will continue, but they will incorporate other health-care elements, including finding the cause of the stroke, starting the recovery process, and preventing stroke recurrence.

Supportive Care

Supportive methods to stabilize the airway, breathing, and circulation of a stroke patient are maintained after the first twenty-four hours. These methods include using a breathing machine if he cannot breathe on his own or protect his airway, providing oxygen via a tube in the nostrils if needed, continuing intravenous fluids, treating fevers, and maintaining normal blood sugar levels.

In addition, several steps are taken to prevent common complications from a stroke. The most common complications are pneumonia, blood clot in the leg (known as deep vein thrombosis, or DVT), urinary tract infection, heart attack, expansion of the stroke, recurrent (or repeat) strokes, and bleeding into an ischemic stroke (i.e., bleeding into the damaged tissue).

In order to prevent pneumonia, it is critical to ensure a patient passes a bedside swallow evaluation before he eats. If he fails the bedside swallow test, a tube may be inserted from the nose into the stomach. Medications, fluids, and nutrition can be supplied via this tube. This tube is temporary. If it looks like it will be needed for longer than two weeks, the tube will likely be removed in favor of a different tube placed directly into the stomach through the abdomen. This is a reversible procedure. A patient's tube can be taken out once he can eat safely and meet his nutritional requirements.

Another common complication is a clot in the leg. As you probably know, blood clots can form in veins in the legs after periods of not moving, such as long plane flights. The same is true in the hospital, when one lies in bed for hours at a time with minimal movement. A low dose of blood-thinning medication given by subcutaneous injection (injection under the skin) can prevent blood clots. Since doctors use only a low dose of blood-thinning medication to prevent leg clots, it can even be given to a patient who has a bleed in the brain—provided the bleed is stable, and two days have elapsed since the bleed first occurred. In addition, *intermittent pneumatic compression* devices may be used. These devices include an inflatable jacket (sleeve, glove, or, most commonly, boot) that encloses the arm or leg. The jacket is connected to an air pump, which fills the chambers of the jacket to pressurize the tissues in the arm or leg. This pressurization causes a release of natural anti-clotting factors, thus reducing the risk of clot formation.

Another common complication is a *urinary tract infection*. The risk of a urinary tract infection increases if there is a catheter in the bladder, so a patient's healthcare team will try to remove it as soon as possible to avoid infection. Urinating in a bedpan or urinal is preferable to keeping a catheter in. There are also less invasive catheters known as condom catheters for men and external catheters for women.

Heart attacks occur after stroke because individuals with atherosclerosis in the arteries to the brain often have atherosclerosis in the arteries of the heart. Occasionally, a heart attack can be the cause of a stroke. For example, if a person has a heart attack, certain muscles of the heart can become damaged, causing it to pump less efficiently. In this scenario, the blood doesn't move the way it normally does, and stagnant blood is prone to forming clots. If a clot forms and then leaves the heart, it can travel to the brain, causing a stroke. More often, however, a heart attack occurs after a stroke. For this reason, a doctor will monitor for signs of damage to the heart using an electrocardiogram (ECG, or EKG) and blood test.

Ischemic strokes can enlarge in the first few days. As mentioned earlier, when there is a blockage of an artery, there is territory that is irreversibly damaged, and a surrounding area that is at risk of dying. There are several strategies to maximize blood flow to this area. A healthcare provider may give her patient antiplatelet medication, such as aspirin. She may administer intravenous fluids. Finally, she may allow his blood pressure to autoregulate on the higher side. Despite these treatments and supportive measures, strokes sometimes expand. If this happens, weakness can worsen or new symptoms can develop, depending on which part of the brain is affected. In connection with the expansion of a patient's stroke, a healthcare team will usually give him more intravenous fluids, suggest keeping him in bed, with the head of the bed at 30 degrees, and even give him medication to increase his blood pressure.

Hemorrhagic strokes typically enlarge in the first twenty-four hours (longer if a blood thinner was being used). The main strategy for preventing a bleed from expanding is lowering a patient's blood pressure and reversing the effects of any blood-thinning medication he might have taken.

Another possibility is the occurrence of a new ischemic stroke in a different area. This situation is rare, but it can occur if there is an unstable plaque in one of the arteries, irregular heart rhythm, or a clot in the heart. This is one of the reasons to keep a patient in the hospital after a stroke, even if his symptoms have improved and he has minimal residual symptoms. The key to preventing another stroke is determining what the underlying cause is. In order to accomplish this task, a patient's healthcare team will conduct several diagnostic studies and check blood tests.

Finally, in strokes caused by a blocked artery, the damaged tissue is prone to bleeding. When bleeding occurs in the area of an ischemic stroke, it is known as "hemorrhagic conversion of an ischemic stroke." If this conversion happens, depending on its severity, blood-thinning medication may need to be put on hold as the healthcare team discusses the pros and cons of using this type of medication in such a situation.

Diagnosis

In order to determine the cause of an ischemic stroke, there are several tests that are typically carried out: imaging of the brain and its arteries, evaluation of the heart, and blood tests. Regarding imaging, if it is not done in the first twenty-four hours, in many cases *magnetic resonance imaging* (MRI) of the brain will be requested. An MRI scan provides a greater level of detail than that offered by a CT scan. In addition to showing where a stroke is located, an MRI gives an indication of the age of a stroke (hours, days, or weeks) and can reveal old strokes—even prior strokes that did not have any symptoms (also known as silent strokes).

In addition, an MRI can provide clues as to whether there is underlying disease of the tiny arteries that supply the brain, and if there are any microbleeds that most commonly occur in the setting of high blood pressure. If a patient's arteries were not evaluated in the first twenty-four hours, imaging will often be performed to look at them. There are several ways to look at arteries, including a *CT angiogram* (a CT with dye injected in a vein), an *MR angiogram* (this can be done with or without dye), an ultrasound, and a conventional angiogram. Different situations call for different imaging modalities. By looking at the arteries, a healthcare team can see if there are any areas of narrowing, blockage, atherosclerotic plaques, or tears in the arteries (dissections). It can also evaluate the network of arteries to see how the blood is rerouting in the presence of a blockage.

In addition to looking for signs of a heart attack with an ECG and blood tests, a healthcare team will usually take a look at the heart with a transthoracic echocardiogram (ultrasound) to search for potential sources of a stroke. This test is usually performed to look for clots in the chambers of the heart (atrium or ventricle), determine how well the heart pumps, and observe the valves. In an individual without any risk factors for stroke, a healthcare team may look for a connection between the left and the right side of his heart, such as a patent foramen ovale (PFO). As mentioned in the previous chapter, a PFO is a passageway between the left atrium and right atrium, and it is present in one out of four people. If a person has a PFO, it means that if he develops a blood clot in the leg, it can travel through his heart to his brain. In someone without a PFO, the clot will go to the lungs.

Since a PFO is relatively common, doctors typically don't look for a PFO in every person who has had a stroke. They tend to look for one if there are no other risk factors for stroke, or if the stroke looks like it came from the heart. In some instances, a different type of ultrasound is required, known as a *transesophageal echocardiogram*. This type of ultrasound is done under sedation and involves putting a camera down the throat to look at the heart. This type of ultrasound offers a better look at certain structures of the heart, including the valves, the *left atrial appendage* (an outpouching of the left atrium), and the aorta, the main artery that supplies blood from the heart to the body.

A healthcare team will also look at the rhythm of a patient's heart to look for signs of an irregular heartbeat (atrial fibrillation). Over the first twenty-four hours in the hospital, a patient will be attached to a cardiac monitor, which will allow his healthcare team to look for an irregular rhythm. If the healthcare team strongly suspects that the stroke is from the heart, then it may suggest long-term monitoring. Luckily there are numerous monitoring options, including a patch that is worn for two weeks at a time and a device that is inserted just under the skin.

The key laboratory tests after stroke include a fasting lipid panel (total cholesterol, low-density lipoprotein cholesterol, high-density lipoprotein cholesterol, and triglycerides), hemoglobin A1c (a measure of blood sugar over the past three months), markers of inflammation, thyroid tests, and occasionally infectious tests (such as syphilis). In some cases, a healthcare team may do other blood tests to look for abnormalities in clotting or conditions where the body's immune system attacks itself.

Treatment and Prevention

As recently mentioned, aspirin is given within the first twenty-four hours of an ischemic stroke. After the first few days, this antiplatelet medication can be switched out for a different antiplatelet such as clopidogrel (Plavix) or a combination of extended-release dipyridamole and aspirin (Aggrenox). In certain circumstances, instead of an antiplatelet, an anticoagulant, which is a stronger blood thinner, will be used. As previously explained, this blood thinner is used in conditions such as a blood clot in the heart or an irregular heart rhythm.

Another key medication to prevent another stroke is a cholesterol medication called a *statin*. There are numerous statins to choose from, but the statin that has been shown to reduce a patient's risk of having another stroke is atorvastatin (Lipitor). In a trial that tested atorvastatin in stroke patients, researchers treated patients who had LDL cholesterol levels above 100 mg/dL and whose strokes were not due to heart conditions with 80 mg of the drug daily. This trial showed that those who took 80 mg of atorvastatin every day were less likely to have another stroke than those who did not. In addition to controlling cholesterol, it is important to control blood sugar with diet and medication, if needed, in order to prevent another stroke.

Finally, the most important risk factor to control is blood pressure. By controlling blood pressure, stroke occurrence could be reduced by half. Therefore, it is important to keep blood pressure at a reading of 130/80 mmHg or less in order to prevent a stroke. The tricky thing, though, is that immediately after a stroke, blood pressure needs to be a little higher to ensure that enough blood flow is getting to the brain. Since it's a delicate balance, a healthcare team will usually start a patient on blood pressure medication after a couple of days and then gently lower his blood pressure. Several weeks after the stroke, it will be more important to get blood pressure into the normal range.

CONCLUSION

During a patient's hospitalization for stroke, his healthcare team will provide supportive care, perform numerous tests to determine a diagnosis, initiate treatment, and start medication to prevent another stroke. The next key step is to start therapy. Therapy is geared towards maintaining range of motion and starting the process of recovery. The next chapter provides information on the process of rehabilitation from stroke.

4

∫troke Rehabilitation

Once a stroke has occurred, how does a patient get back to his old life when faced with new limitations? As discussed in Chapter 1, stroke effects can vary from individual to individual. As explained in Chapter 2, functions that may be affected depend on several factors. The location within the brain where a stroke occurs is important. The size of a stroke is also relevant—a large stroke can affect more functions than a smaller one in the same area. Even a small stroke, however, can have a profound impact if it affects key areas of the brain. In addition the time it takes to get to the hospital and receive treatment is of great relevance. For each minute the brain is deprived of oxygen, 1.9 million neurons (nerve cells), 14 billion synapses (connections between nerve cells), and 12 km (7.5 miles) of myelinated fibers (the cell parts that work like electrical wires transmitting signals) are destroyed. Finally, each individual's vascular network influences the physical deficits brought about by a stroke. A person with a robust network of blood vessels to the brain may have a better outcome than someone with numerous blockages of his blood vessels.

Since stroke symptoms depend on the above-referenced factors, each stroke survivor will have unique rehabilitation needs. One stroke survivor may have primarily muscle weakness and balance issues, while another may have trouble speaking and understanding what is being said. Once the effects of a stroke have been evaluated, rehabilitation therapies will be tailored specifically to the survivor's needs. There is no one-size-fits-all approach.

As mentioned in Chapter 1, neuroplasticity refers to the brain's ability to reorganize itself in response to changes in behavioral demands. The amazing thing is that neuroplasticity is always active—in the healthy as well as the damaged brain. By using the brain's innate neuroplasticity, a survivor can facilitate recovery from a stroke. As a result of neuroplasticity, although nerve networks have been damaged, the brain can create new pathways and regain functions that seemed lost. Imagine there's an accident on the freeway and the freeway is shut down. One can take side streets to avoid the blockage. If side streets are not available, new ones can be created over time. Neuroplasticity works by recruiting non-affected parts of the brain and reorganizing nerve networks.

Some stroke survivors with severe disabilities initially can improve dramatically. A small percentage of stroke survivors, about 10 percent, recover almost completely, while 25 percent recover with minor impairments. The process is long and typically takes months. Given the brain's ability to form new networks, there's no time limit to recovery, although the most dramatic improvements will be in the first weeks or months. Some individuals continue therapy for years.

WHAT IS REHABILITATION?

Rehabilitation is the process in which stroke survivors work on restoring their bodies and brains so that they can either return to their former lives or develop new, meaningful, and fulfilling new lives. These therapies can be grueling. In an inpatient rehabilitation unit, therapists aim for three hours of therapy a day. Therapy is normally carried out in both the morning and afternoon, with time out for lunch and rest. Each therapy session can be exhausting, so it's important to rest when possible. Injured brain cells need time to repair themselves, old neural pathways need time to reroute themselves from injured areas to other parts of the brain, and new brain cells need time to grow. At night, sleep strengthens and organizes memories of the previous day, helping people learn.

Repetition

Remember the old saying "practice makes perfect"? This is certainly true of rehabilitation. During the course of rehabilitation, a therapist will work with a patient on movements that serve a particular function. Examples include grasping and using a spoon, picking up objects, opening and closing a jar, throwing a ball, bathing, getting dressed, grooming, going to the toilet, and walking. The key to a patient's improvement is his repetition of these movements. It is more impactful in recovery to practice movements that are needed to perform day-to-day activities than to focus on strength training, such as lifting weights. The connections between a person's brain and muscles are organized according to specific tasks, not by particular muscles. In addition, the brain reorganizes better when tasks are meaningful to the person doing them. Repetition alone, without usefulness or meaning in terms of function, has a weaker effect on recovery.

Constraining One Limb

In some cases, a therapist may suggest immobilizing a patient's unaffected arm. This is called *constraint-induced movement therapy* (CIMT). In CIMT, a patient's unaffected (or less affected) limb is put in a mitt or sling in order to encourage his affected limb to attempt particular movements.

In some trials, researchers constrained subjects less affected arms for up to 90 percent of waking hours for fourteen days. A modified version of CIMT constrains a patient's less affected arm for one hour a day, three days a week, for ten weeks. It is important for a patient to use his affected arm outside therapy as much as possible and understand how to do so. CIMT is most effective an individual with at least some movement in his weak arm.

Additional Strategies

There are numerous additional strategies a patient can use to encourage the return of normal movement. Strengthening upper extremity muscles with light weights can be helpful when done in addition to task-specific training. Exercises should be recommended by a therapist and done in normal movement patterns; otherwise, individuals may reinforce abnormal movement patterns and cause damage to muscles and tendons. In addition, once abnormal patterns are "wired in," it is hard to retrain the brain to do normal movement patterns. In patients who have only minimal movement in their arms, robotic and biofeedback therapies can help with movement practice. There are different types of robots, including workstation devices that are used in rehabilitation facilities and wearable exoskeleton devices that can be used at home. A review of numerous clinical trials showed that upper limb robotic therapy can improve activities of daily living and arm function.

Neuromuscular electrical stimulation can be used in individuals who are capable of only minimal muscle contraction. This therapy involves applying an electrical stimulus to a muscle, which causes it to contract. It strengthens the connection between the brain and the muscle and is most effective when used with task-specific training. It can also be used to prevent muscle wasting or provide range of motion. When used for six hours a day, it has been shown to aid in the prevention or correction of partial dislocation of the shoulder joint, which is a common complication after stroke in individuals with paralysis or severe arm weakness.

Imagining doing tasks without doing them, called *mental imagery,* is beneficial when added to upper extremity exercises and functional activities. While this is typically taught in a therapy session, it is help-ful to use it when practicing functional movements. In mental practice studies, participants listened to an audio of different functional tasks (e.g., turning pages in a book, combing hair, taking a drink), imagined performing those tasks without doing them, and then worked on the tasks in therapy. Videos are available online with guidance of mental practice of functional tasks. Virtual reality and video games may have the potential to impact motor learning, but studies thus far have been small and results have been inconsistent.

Stimulation of the brain through the use of magnets or currents (i.e., transcranial magnetic stimulation and transcranial direct cur-rent stimulation) is being studied as an approach for maximizing the learning of movements and preventing the muscles from becoming tight and frozen. *Transcranial magnetic stimulation* (TMS) involves the use of magnetic fields to stimulate nerve cells in the brain. During a TMS session, an electromagnetic coil is placed against the scalp. The electromagnet painlessly delivers a magnetic pulse that stimulates nerve cells. TMS has been effective in treating depression, but its effect on stroke recovery is still being studied. In *transcranial direct current stimulation,* two electrodes are placed over the head. These electrodes provide painless electrical stimulation that either excites or blocks nerve activity. Several studies suggest that this therapy may be effective in stroke recovery, but it is still under investigation.

Advice for Caregivers
ACT AS A GATE KEEPER

If you are the caregiver of a stroke survivor who is in rehabilitation, you can act as a gate keeper. Give relatives and friends specific times to visit that will work with his therapy schedule while also providing time for rest. Tell visitors that he gets tired easily, so short visits—five minutes at the beginning—would be appreciated. Make sure only people he wants to see are given permission to see him.

PREVENTING AND ADDRESSING COMPLICATIONS

In addition to enhancing recovery, it is essential to take precautions to prevent complications after stroke. Some of these complications, such as a blood clot in the legs and pneumonia have been mentioned earlier in Chapter 3. In this chapter, we will address a few additional complications and steps to avoid them.

Prevention of Skin Breakdown

After a stroke, patients typically do not move as much as they used to, and may have numbness in their arms or legs. As a result, their skin can become irritated and develop sores or ulcers. Strategies to reduce skin irritation include frequent turning if confined to a bed (at least every two hours), checking skin daily, engaging in good hygiene, using a special mattress and proper wheelchair seating, eliminating friction, minimizing pressure, providing appropriate support surfaces, avoiding excessive moisture, and maintaining adequate nutrition and hydration.

Prevention of Contractures

After a stroke that affects strength on one side, approximately 60 percent of patients develop contractures within the first year. A *contracture* is a tightening or shortening of muscles, causing joint stiffness, and difficulty moving. Contractures occur when muscles are inactive, and elastic tissues are replaced by rigid tissues. Contractures prevent joints from moving freely. For example, an elbow contracture can make it painful and difficult to straighten the arm. A wrist contracture can make it difficult to lift the hand. In the setting of a stroke, the flexors in the arm are usually stronger than the extensors, so contractures are more likely to occur in the flexed position. The opposite pattern is seen in the leg, with the extensors being stronger than the flexors. If you see someone with a stroke with weakness on one side, you may notice that his elbow, wrist, and fingers are bent, while his leg is straight on the affected side.

Wrist contractures are most often seen in those who do not recover the ability to use the hand. Contractures can cause pain and make it difficult to perform self-care, including dressing and hygiene. Clinicians often recommend daily stretching of the weak limbs at each joint to avoid contracture development.

The use of arm splints to prevent contractures is controversial. While some organizations recommend them, others advise against them, given the limited research on their effectiveness. On the other hand, use of an ankle splint is generally recommended. The ankle splint keeps the ankle at 90 degrees (after a stroke, the foot normally points down because the ability to lift the foot up is impaired). Positioning is important too. Early after stroke, positioning the weak shoulder in external rotation for 30 minutes each day can help prevent shoulder contractures.

Spasticity

Spasticity—continual contraction of the muscles—is also common after stroke. Normally, the brain and spinal cord send two types of signals to muscles—*excitatory signals* to contract and *inhibitory signals* to relax. In the setting of a stroke, the inhibitory signals may be damaged, resulting in continuous excitation of the muscle, and stiff, tight, painful muscles.

Shoulder Pain

Shoulder pain is common after stroke, affecting up to 20 percent of patients in the first year. It is often associated with shoulder *subluxation* and weakness of the arm. A shoulder subluxation is a partial dislocation of the shoulder joint. This occurs when the ball of the upper arm bone (i.e., the humerus) partly comes out of the socket that holds it. The shoulder is the most mobile joint in the body. Most of the stability of this joint is provided by the muscles. When these muscles become weak after a stroke, the stability is compromised, and the ball of the humerus can move from its normal position in the socket and become partially dislocated (i.e., subluxed).

Spasticity can also contribute to shoulder pain. Additionally, patients with stroke affecting arm strength can develop tissue injury, including accumulation of fluid in the shoulder, inflammation of the tendons, and tears in the muscles stabilizing the shoulder (i.e., rotator cuff muscles). Stroke can also affect the pain pathways of the brain, causing changes in pain thresholds.

Strategies to prevent and treat shoulder pain include proper positioning, maintaining range of motion at the shoulder, and training to improve movements. For those in wheelchairs, lap trays and arm troughs can reduce shoulder pain and subluxation. Some clinicians recommend passive range of motion exercises. The use of arm slings, particularly during walking can be used as well. Other techniques such as strapping or taping the shoulder, acupuncture, and electrical stimulation have been studied with variable results. At this time there is insufficient evidence for shoulder strapping or taping. Acupuncture has shown positive results in small studies. Skin surface electrical stimulation has also been studied and shown inconsistent results.

Corticosteroid injections in the shoulder joint can be used to treat shoulder pain, although related studies have shown conflicting results on their benefits. Botulinum toxin injections into the shoulder muscles have shown mixed results as well. Nerve blocks, on the other hand, have been shown to help reduce pain for up to twelve weeks after treatment. Finally, medications to address nerve pain can be used.

Fall Prevention

Up to 70 percent of stroke survivors fall during the first 6 months after discharge from the hospital or rehabilitation facility. Stroke can affect balance, strength, coordination, sensation, and vision, making stroke survivors prone to falling. Fear of falling can be dangerous—resulting in decreased activity, deconditioning, limited mobility, loss of independence, social isolation, and depression. It is therefore critical to address fall prevention strategies early. Strategies to reduce falls include participating in exercise programs with balance training, formal fall prevention programs in the hospital, tai chi training, and making changes to the house to avoid falls. It is essential to remove hazards in the house; this includes removing boxes, electrical cords, and phone cords from walkways; moving coffee tables, magazine racks, and plants from high-traffic areas; securing loose rugs with double-faced tape, tacks, or slip-resistant backing (or removing loose rugs from walkways); repairing loose wooden floorboards and carpeting; storing dishes, clothing, food, and other necessities within easy reach; cleaning spills; and using non-slip mats in the bathtub or shower.

The home should be brightly lit in order to avoid tripping on objects that are hard to see. It is helpful to place nightlights in bedrooms, bathrooms, and hallways; place a lamp within reach of the bed; turn on lights before going up or down the stairs; and store flashlights in easy-to-find places in case of power outages. Assistance devices in the home may be helpful too: handrails for both sides of the stairways; grab bars for the shower or tub; and a plastic seat for the shower or tub. An occupational therapist can provide information about home safety.

THERAPY TEAM

Stroke survivors are cared for by a team of experts who work together to come up with the best treatments for these patients. These occupational, physical, and speech therapists are discussed in great detail in the next three chapters, but here are brief, simple descriptions of these healthcare providers. The goals of therapists in an inpatient setting are to evaluate how a patient functions; jump-start the process of recovery; determine the safest place for a patient to go—whether it is home, a long-term rehabilitation facility, nursing facility, or board and care—and ensure that he can safely go to this place.

Registered Nurse (RN)

Registered nurses (RNs) obtain their degrees after finishing a two-year associate's degree program in nursing or a four-year bachelor's degree program in nursing. Some RNs may also have a master's degree in nursing, which allows them to specialize in a particular area or take the first step in achieving a nursing degree at the doctoral level. The duties of an RN include administering medicine or other forms of treatment, operating and monitoring medical equipment, preparing patients for exams, making assessments, collaborating with supervising physicians, teaching patients how to manage medical conditions, recording patients' symptoms and medical histories, and overseeing the work of licensed practical nurses and licensed vocational nurses.

Licensed Practical Nurse (LPN) and Licensed Vocational Nurse (LVN)

Licensed practical nurses and *licensed vocational nurses* receive their credentials by completing a state-approved training program, which results in either a diploma, certificate, or associate's degree. The majority of these programs can be completed in one year, although some offer an extensive nursing curriculum and may take longer. These nurses typically monitor a patient's vital signs (such as heart rate, blood pressure, and respiratory rate), administer basic care, and report concerns to registered nurses and physicians. They may help patients with bathing and toileting, and they aid in transferring patients from bed to wheelchair.

Medical Assistant

Medical assistants work with the healthcare team. Like LPNs and LVNs, they are trained to take vital signs, administer basic care, and report any concerns to registered nurses and physicians. They are also able to help with bathing, toileting, and transferring patients in the hospital.

Doctor

Patients in rehabilitation are taken care of by specially trained doctors, not by primary care doctors. These physicians may be experts in emergency medicine, neurology (the study of the brain and nerves), or physical medicine and rehabilitation.

Nurse Practitioner and Physician Assistant

Many hospitals also use *nurse practitioners* and *physician assistants*, collectively called *advanced practice providers*. These clinicians are not physicians, but they are able to do many of the tasks physicians do. A nurse must undergo additional training after getting a bachelor's degree and master's degree in nursing in order to gain a nurse practitioner degree. Nurse practitioners are able to treat patients independently and prescribe medications, working under their own licenses. Similarly, a physician assistant degree may be acquired with additional training after a bachelor's degree. Physician assistants are able to treat patients and prescribe medications, but they may do so only under the authority of a physician.

Occupational Therapist

Occupational therapy (OT) is aimed at enabling stroke survivors to participate in the activities that they need or want to do. An *occupational therapist,* also called an OT, focuses on a stroke survivor's motor, cognitive, and psychological impairments that limit his ability to engage in activities, including social participation. Initially, an OT may focus on activities of daily living such as eating, bathing, dressing, going to the bathroom, and moving from bed to wheelchair (and vice versa). Over time, the focus will shift to how a survivor can engage better in his family life, home, community, and profession.

Physical Therapist

Physical therapy (PT) addresses the ability to move, reduce pain, restore functional movement, and prevent physical disability. *Physical therapists,* also called PTs, generally help with walking and balance, and often provide exercises for strength and range of motion of affected limbs.

Speech Therapist

Known also as a *speech-language pathologist* (SLP), a *speech therapist* (ST) addresses three main areas: swallowing, speech, and cognition (the ability to think and process information). She first assesses swallowing function after stroke. In relation to strokes, survivors can have difficulty chewing and swallowing. If this occurs, there's a risk of *aspiration* (i.e., food or liquid going down the breathing pipe). If a stroke survivor aspirates, an infection of the lungs, pneumonia, can develop. This is why it is critical for a speech therapist to check swallowing after a stroke. Second, a speech therapist addresses communication needs, including speech, the ability to understand others, and the ability to read and write. Finally, she addresses a patient's ability to think and process information.

AUXILIARY TEAM MEMBERS

In addition to the main stroke rehabilitation team members, there are other personnel who assist stroke survivors during rehabilitation. A stroke patient and his family should get to know these people and appreciate how they can help survivors and their families by answering questions and addressing special needs.

Social Worker

A *social worker* is an expert who is trained to help a patient, his family, and his friends cope with the new problems that arise in the aftermath of a stroke. Social workers will inquire about a patient's support system to determine what he will need after discharge from the hospital.

If a stroke survivor is scheduled to go home, a social worker will determine and discuss what changes need to be made to the home to accommodate his needs. A social worker may ask about a survivor's financial situation in order to provide him and his family with valuable resources such as assistance with food programs, disability insurance, and social security. This team member can help navigate private health insurance or government insurance such as Medicaid or Medicare. Finally, a social worker is there to provide support to a stroke survivor's family, caregivers, and friends.

Case Manager

A *case manager* works with the entire healthcare team to address the medical, physical, emotional, financial, psychosocial, and behavioral needs of a patient. She often works with health insurance plans, government agencies, and employers to ensure services are received. A case manager's process involves nine phases which span the continuum of care from emergency department through rehabilitation and recovery: screening, assessing, stratifying risk, planning, care coordination, follow-up, assisting with transitions, communicating transitions, and evaluation. You can expect a case manager to act as an advocate throughout the entire sequence of care. There is some overlap between the role of case manager and social worker. Indeed, some hospitals do not have case managers at all.

Registered Dietitian

A *registered dietitian* (RD) may visit a stroke patient several times. This person is highly trained in the science of nutrition and has studied at length the specific nutritional needs of someone who has had a stroke or has other special medical needs. If a patient is receiving tube feeding, a dietitian will advise the care team on the best combination of nutrients for recovery.

An RD can be involved in advising a stroke survivor on how to change his diet to regain health and prevent another stroke. As the old saying goes, an ounce of prevention is worth a pound of cure. The importance of this change in diet cannot be overstated. Part IV provides education on nutrition, explaining what to avoid, what to eat, and how to plan simple, delicious, and highly nutritious meals. (See page 233.)

Spiritual Care Team

The spiritual care team refers to all the people who have been ordained for religious duties. A spiritual team member employed by the hospital or rehabilitation unit will drop by to see a patient, if needed, to help with spiritual needs and provide comfort, peace, and optimism. A patient does not need to have been religious before the stroke. A stroke survivor can request a spiritual team member to visit at any time if he is feeling afraid, depressed, or worried. A spiritual team member can also help a patient's family deal with this new situation, as a stroke can change the lives of everyone involved.

If a patient has a church, synagogue, mosque, or other institution that he normally attends, the hospital can contact this place of worship to arrange a visit. When necessary, volunteers from these houses of worship may be able to help when a stroke survivor leaves the facility by driving him to appointments, providing meals, or dropping by for a visit to brighten his day. Stroke survivors need all the help and support they can get.

REHABILITATION BEGINS IN ACUTE CARE

Once a patient has been stabilized in an acute care setting and is out of immediate danger, rehabilitation can start between twenty-four and forty-eight hours after his stroke. Rehabilitation needs are assessed as soon as possible while a patient is still in bed, where physical, mental, and language abilities are tested by the doctor and therapists to see how extensive his stroke was.

Stroke survivors are visited by various therapists—speech, occupational, and physical— who test their abilities to speak, understand, swallow, perform their activities of daily living, and move. These tests also act as initial therapies. For example, if a patient has weakness or paralysis on the left side, a physical therapist can help him move his left arm and leg, or even move them for him. Movement is important to retain range of motion, so muscles don't get stuck in one position, and to rewire the brain, restoring connections with muscles.

Evaluation and therapy in acute care begins in bed. A doctor and therapist will want a patient to move his arms and legs to retain range of motion, move around the bed, roll over, and sit up. These exercises are not easy for many stroke survivors and, when achieved, are major victories. Patients are instructed to practice bending and straightening their arms, hands, and fingers; and their legs, feet, and toes. If these are difficult motions for a patient to make, a therapist will help him with these tasks. The sooner a patient can move around, the better for his brain and muscles, and their ability to work together, even if it means a therapist moving his limbs on his behalf.

As soon as possible, acute care staff will want a stroke patient sitting up on the side of his bed, standing briefly, and then moving to a chair. He may feel weak, but it will feel good to be out of bed. The risk of pneumonia is high in a new stroke patient, but it decreases if he doesn't lie in bed all day. A stroke survivor may be exhausted after what seems like a minor activity, but getting up and about is necessary if he wishes to gain strength, endurance, and prevent other medical conditions from taking hold.

Bedside activities include a patient washing his face, brushing his teeth, combing his hair, sitting on the edge of the bed, and eating a meal—this is all therapy. If needed, a nurse, nurse's aide, or therapist will help him. He may also need assistance in picking up and using kitchen utensils, pouring liquids, or drinking from a glass. Getting food or beverages to his mouth could be challenging. If a patient has trouble swallowing, a speech therapist will advise on the consistency of food required to avoid aspiration.

For bathroom needs, a stroke survivor may use a bedpan initially, progress to a bedside commode, and finally move to the bathroom with the help of an aide or therapist if needed.

LEAVING ACUTE CARE

A stay in acute care can last days or even weeks. Stroke patients are typically admitted to intensive care units (ICUs), step-down units (one level below ICUs), or telemetry units (one level below step-down units). After a patient's diagnostic evaluation is complete and he is medically stable, a rehabilitation team will determine if a stay in an "acute rehabilitation" facility would be appropriate.

When outpatient therapy is prescribed, a patient typically returns to see therapists in outpatient therapy gyms. The healthcare team will recommend sites for rehabilitation, and his family and friends can help choose a rehabilitation site that is best for him. Family or friends may want to visit two or three facilities on a patient's behalf. Since the qualities of various rehabilitation centers can vary greatly, it is important to ask the right questions and look around carefully. When decided on a rehabilitation facility, the following criteria should be considered:

- What services does the facility offer?

- Are there opportunities to do exercises and use exercise equipment outside of therapy sessions?

- Is there a therapy group a patient can attend?

- Do patients get therapy every day, including weekends?

- Are meals supervised by a registered dietitian?

- Is the facility clean and well kept?

- Does the staff seem caring and upbeat?

- Is the location of the facility close enough so that friends and family can visit easily?

- What do other stroke patients and their families think about the facility?

- What are the costs involved, including those for check-ups and drug administration?

- How much of the total cost will be covered by insurance?

Beyond any immediate search for a rehabilitation center, a patient's healthcare provider may have a rehabilitation unit she favors. She may also be able to give him a general idea of how long he will stay there, and whether or not he will be able to return home or need to arrange some other temporary or permanent living situation. A survivor's length of stay will depend, in part, on how severe his stroke was, how much progress he is making, and how diligently he dedicates himself to the therapy.

The average length of stay in an inpatient rehabilitation facility is fourteen days. A patient and his family should not expect full recovery in this time. The purpose of this rehabilitation stay is to evaluate a patient, teach him and his family the exercises he should do, accelerate his recovery process, teach his caregivers safe ways to assist him, and ensure a safe discharge to his next living space, whether it's his home or a long-term facility.

If a patient is too weak or tired to participate in inpatient rehabilitation, or if his deficits are mild, therapists may recommend a less intense program. If a patient goes home, therapists may recommend outpatient therapy, in which the patient would attend therapy gym sessions of thirty minutes to one hour. If a patient is discharged to a long-term acute care facility (a step down from acute inpatient rehabilitation) or a skilled nursing facility, this facility will likely provide therapy on a less frequent basis.

CONCLUSION

At this point, you should have a better understanding of what rehabilitation is, and of the different professionals who attend to a stroke survivor in the ICU and later in rehabilitation. It is important to emphasize that all these professionals work as a team to get a patient better as soon as possible. They communicate daily with each other and have meetings about a patient's changing needs. The next few chapters provide more detailed descriptions of individual rehabilitation therapies, including occupational, physical, and speech therapies.

5

Occupational Therapy

As you learned in the last chapter, occupational therapy—OT for short, which may stand for "occupational therapy" or "occupational therapist"—is one important piece of the recovery puzzle. So, what exactly is occupational therapy and why is it important? OT helps patients perform activities of daily living, recover purposeful movement, and return to work. "Activities of daily living" include basic self-care tasks such as eating, bathing, dressing, toileting, and grooming. More complex activities of daily living include managing finances, handling transportation, shopping, preparing meals (e.g., putting away groceries, using a stove safely, and placing food on plates), using a telephone or computer, managing medications, doing laundry (e.g., washing and drying clothes, folding them, and placing them where they belong), housework, and basic home maintenance.

After a stroke, a patient will likely experience multiple challenges. In OT, the term "occupational" refers to much more than what may be associated with an individual's occupation. It refers to all the daily activities a stroke survivor needs, wants, and enjoys doing.

If a patient is having trouble moving and coordinating his hands and fingers, an OT will use various exercises to help him relearn these skills. If a patient wishes to return to driving, an OT will work on the skills needed for him to drive safely. If a patient needs to return to the workplace, an OT will help him regain any pertinent skills he has lost, such as typing or using small tools. If the acts of lifting and carrying are a problem, these will be addressed by either occupational therapy or physical therapy, also known as PT.

So, what is the difference between OT and PT? Occupational therapists work on motor function and coordination needed to do specified activities, often in the upper extremities and trunk. Physical therapists work on motor function, too, but their work is primarily related to mobility and transfers (moving from sitting to standing or from one seated position to another). While PTs address balance as it relates to mobility, OTs address balance through functional activities, such as standing at a sink to groom oneself or moving about a kitchen to prepare a meal. Physical therapists and occupational therapists work with and consult each other during a patient's rehabilitation. They read each other's notes and communicate with the doctor who oversees the rehabilitation team. Occupational and physical therapists often coordinate their efforts when developing goals with a patient in order to maximize his rehabilitation potential.

Occupational therapists are highly educated and experienced professionals. In order to be certified, an OT must have a master's degree or doctorate in occupational therapy. She must complete an internship and be certified by a national board. Occupational therapists help people of all ages live more active lives with injury, illnesses such as a stroke, or any type of disability.

SETTING GOALS

An OT works not only with a patient but also his healthcare providers, physical therapist, speech therapist, and perhaps even his social worker to make a list of his short-term and long-term goals. For example, a patient's primary goal may be to take care of himself if he lives alone, or to be able to return to work part-time, or to be able to play cards or throw balls with his grandchildren, or perhaps to dance or sway to music he loves. An OT will ask targeted questions to help her patient set goals for his therapy.

Work Skills

If a patient will be returning to his job after his recovery, his OT (and his PT) will want to know about his work and the exact physical and cognitive tasks he performs there. An OT will review the functions that a patient may need to work on. An occupational therapist will break down tasks into smaller steps and skills to identify specific problem areas for a patient. These problem areas will become treatment goals.

An OT will likely ask a patient several questions. Does he expect to return to work? If so, does he hope to return to work on a full-time or part-time basis? What are the skills he will need to accomplish this goal? How is his workplace laid out? Are there stairs or an elevator? Will he spend most of his day sitting, standing, or walking? How will he be using his hands? Can he possibly work from home on some days? If his speech is affected, how much will his job involve speaking? A speech therapist will help him with speech and language problems.

Living Arrangements

A patient's OT will want to know about his previous living arrangements and future living plans. An OT will help ensure a patient's safe and smooth transition from inpatient rehabilitation to a more permanent living space (or from one living arrangement to another) by recommending durable medical equipment (such as wheelchairs, walkers, hospital beds, and shower chairs). Does a patient have stairs or other challenges in his house? Does he live alone or with a spouse or other family members? Does he have friends, neighbors, or family nearby to help? Does he have children, grandchildren, or parent, or pets to care for?

Basic Activities of Daily Living

Basic activities of daily living include self-care tasks such as eating, bathing, dressing, grooming, toileting, and mobility. An OT will assess a patient's ability to pick up a fork, use it to pick up food, and bring it to his mouth. She will determine if he can stand in the shower, turn it on, bathe, dry himself, put on clothes, button his shirts, and tie his shoes. She will see if he can brush his teeth, brush his hair, and shave. She will determine if he can walk to the toilet, clean himself, and get back up. These activities are usually done without a second thought, but they often become much more difficult after a stroke and are typically the first things an OT focuses on.

Complex Activities of Daily Living

In addition to addressing basic care activities, OTs help patients perform complex activities related to preparing meals, maintaining a home, and tending to tasks outside the home. An OT will ask her patient numerous questions about these more complex tasks, also called instrumental activities of daily living.

Before a patient had a stroke, did he prepare his own meals, do his own housekeeping, wash and fold his clothes, and so on? Did he drive a car before the stroke? Did he do his own grocery shopping? Did he take himself to the doctor and manage his medications? Is there anyone who could help him with some of these activities either temporarily or permanently—such as hired help or a spouse, family member, or friend?

Leisure Activities

Leisure is important for life balance. An OT will want to know if a patient had any hobbies prior to his stroke. What gave him great pleasure? Did he like to play sports—tennis, golf, swimming, or jogging? Did he love to dance? Did he enjoy long walks or hiking? Did he work out? Did he like to fix things? Did he go out to dinner with friends and family?

Did he enjoy any quiet activities? Was he involved in yoga or tai chi? Did he like to read, do puzzles, knit, watch TV, or play cards or board games with friends or family? Did he like to listen to music? Knowing which activities he enjoyed before his stroke will help his OT (and other therapists) not only to know him better but also to determine which activities may be a good fit for him in the future.

Sex and Intimacy

A patient's OT can also help him in addressing sex and intimacy questions. It is an important topic that often gets left out because it can be uncomfortable to discuss. Some things his OT may discuss following a stroke include safe positions during sex, how to communicate his needs and wants with his partner effectively, how intimacy may be different after a stroke for both parties, and how to achieve intimacy after a stroke.

Advice for Caregivers
ATTENDING OT SESSIONS

If you can, go to some or all OT sessions with your loved one. Doing so will allow you to observe the types of problems your loved one is facing that may not have been obvious to you from simply observing him at rest. It will also enable you to observe how the therapist assists him so that later on you can help him function more independently and do his exercises at home. Your presence in OT sessions will also allow him to see you root for him. If he achieves something he hasn't been able to do, he will see you cheer for him. You can compliment him on each new accomplishment and remark upon how he has improved over the day or week before. Lastly, being there at OT sessions will permit you to ask the therapist questions about anything you or your loved one may not understand. Your input will be valuable to both your loved one and his therapist.

OCCUPATIONAL THERAPY EVALUATION

A variety of therapeutic activities are employed during the course of OT sessions. OT starts in a patient's hospital bed, as described in the previous chapter. As he makes progress, he will be taken to a sink for grooming, a shower for bathing, and eventually the OT room, where he will engage in different activities. He may be amazed at the types of gadgets, machines, and computers his therapists have to assist him. In order to determine the appropriate tools to use, his OT will evaluate numerous issues, including:

- Does he have weakness or numbness?

- Does he need a wheelchair, walker, or cane?

- Has his balance been affected? Does he experience dizziness or feel like he is going to fall?

- How are his fine motor skills in relation to his fingers and hands? Does he have trouble grasping or holding on to things? Does he have trouble making his fingers do what he wants them to do?

- Is his stamina or endurance less than before his stroke? Does he become fatigued quickly?

- Has his vision changed since the stroke? Are there blind spots, double vision, or perceptual difficulties?

- Does he need a bedside commode, shower chair, or adaptive equipment to assist with toileting, bathing, dressing, or meal preparation?

- How are his memory, thinking, attention, language, and math-processing skills?

- Has his mood changed since his stroke? Is he less interested in things that used to interest him? Does he have difficulty coping with the situation he finds himself in after the stroke?

An OT will evaluate a patient to determine what has been affected by a stroke. She will give him tasks to perform, which will allow his healthcare team to tailor his therapies and track his progress. If he is given tasks that require standing, his therapist may put a safety belt around his waist to keep him from falling. Therapists have been trained to keep a patient steady, whether he weighs one hundred pounds or three hundred pounds. The information obtained from these evaluations will likely be forwarded to the patient's health insurance provider. The progress shown on therapy evaluations will determine the coverage provided by his health insurance provider.

Occupational Therapy Tests

An OT may conduct tests on upper extremity movement and sensation, performance on basic and complex activities of daily living, cognition, vision, work, leisure, and sleep. As mentioned, a stroke patient will probably be tested many times throughout OT to assess his progress. Just doing these tests is therapeutic. Eventually, a patient's therapist may be able to show him colorful graphs that dramatically illustrate his progress. His therapist will show him how his scores compare with his previous scores and with those of other patients his age. These scores will show him how much progress he has made and reassure him that his hard work is paying off. If some scores have not improved, his therapist may choose other tasks to accomplish the same goal.

Tests of Activities of Daily Living

An OT may perform standardized tests to evaluate basic tasks of eating, bathing, dressing, grooming, toileting, and mobility. In most cases, they will have a patient perform these various tasks, and help them throughout the process. By watching him perform these tasks, his therapist can determine what assistance is needed, what to work on, and if any assistive equipment is required.

Tests of Fine Motor Skills

Occupational therapists will also assess *fine motor skills,* which are defined as the abilities of the small muscles in the fingers, hands, and wrists to do various activities. These activities include picking up objects and putting them down, tapping fingers, or snapping fingers. Of course, more complicated activities like playing the piano, knitting, or keyboarding require more complex fine motor skills.

An OT may do the following tests to evaluate a patient's fine motor skills: Can he touch his thumb to each of his other fingers? Can he pick up small blocks and put them into a box? How many coins can he pick up off the table and put into a cup in one minute? How many pegs can he put in a pegboard in one minute? A therapist will test both the right hand and the left with each exercise. A patient will do much better when using the hand unaffected by the stroke. Sometimes both sides of the body have been affected by a stroke, however, and so both sides may react more slowly than before.

A stroke patient may find these tasks difficult, but he shouldn't get discouraged. He should tell himself, "I'm going to beat this! I can do this." That's the whole point of therapy: to help stroke survivors regain the skills they had before. Rome wasn't built in a day, and stroke patients will not reacquire lost skills instantly, but they should notice improvement over time, which should make them feel excited and even more determined.

Cognitive Tests

A therapist may also perform tests to measure a patient's attention, language skills, processing time, memory, reasoning skills, and decision-making. For example, a patient may be asked to draw a clock, put the numbers on the face, and draw hands to show a particular time, or to trace his way through a maze. He may be asked to name as many words as he can that start with a particular letter in a given amount of time, or he may be asked to spell a word backwards—for example, "world": D-L-R-O-W.

Advice for Caregivers
PRACTICING MIND TESTS

Mental stimulation is so important in healing the brain. After your loved one has rested, he can practice a few mind tests. He may be able to do simple crossword puzzles, Sudoku, or other puzzles. There are many gaming applications available on smart phones and computers to help stimulate the brain. For example, Lumosity is a free app that offers games designed to improve memory, cognitive ability, and problem-solving skills. It is important to help your loved one exercise his mind, but keep in mind that he may now find it surprising, frustrating, and tiring that tasks he once excelled at are now a challenge. Just keep him practicing.

He may be shown a picture of a shape, told to remember it, and then instructed to find it on a page of several different shapes. His therapist may say a sentence and then ask him to repeat it back to her word for word. All these tests measure his abilities to pay attention, remember things, think things through, make the proper connections from his eyes and ears to his brain, and send the right signals from his brain to his mouth and hands. The brain and its abilities to understand and respond are amazing and complicated. The key to improving them is repetition and practice. If a patient does not understand why he is performing a certain task, he should ask his therapist to explain the reason for doing this task.

Occupational therapists may also evaluate a patient's cognitive abilities during functional activities that require multiple sequential steps and safety precautions, such as preparing a snack in a microwave, making tea on a stovetop, baking brownies, making a call for a specific need, money management at a store or online, or planning transportation.

Vision

An OT may test a patient's vision to see if he has developed visual problems since having a stroke. Of course, a stroke survivor may already be aware that his vision has changed dramatically. This can be disturbing and challenging. The change is determined by the site of the damage to the brain. Some examples of the possible visual problems caused by a stroke include trouble seeing half (either the left or right side) of the visual field, double vision, and difficulty interpreting what is seen.

Advice for Caregivers
VISION PROBLEMS

After his stroke, your loved one may have mild to severe vision problems relating to perception, field of vision, or double vision. Ask his doctor how to categorize these vision problems so that you can find a website that shows how things look to those with this particular problem. The American Stroke Association's website, for example, contains pictures of visual disturbances. (See page 286 of the Resources.) Seeing the problem for yourself may give you more appreciation for the challenge he is facing. Some OTs may recommend a patient visit an optometrist (but not an ophthalmologist, as an ophthalmologist may diagnose visual deficits but do not treat vision problems associated with stroke.) An optometrist may suggest a patient wear prism glasses, which can help the brain recover. Ask your loved one's OT if there are any exercises he could do to improve his visual problems.

Reaction Time

A patient's therapist may test his reaction time. *Reaction time* is the length of time between first seeing or hearing something and reacting to it. For example, the length of time it takes a person to react to a phone ringing or being asked a question. If a patient's reaction time is too long, his OT will suggest exercises to reduce it.

OCCUPATIONAL THERAPY EXERCISES AND ACTIVITIES

A patient's rehabilitation unit may have many important features. For example, it may have a small kitchen and laundry room where he can prepare meals and wash, dry, and fold his clothes. It may have a special bathroom that has stroke-friendly features—a special handheld shower hose, a seat to sit on when the patient is tired, and a non-skid floor. At first, a patient's OT or nurse's aide will help him undertake these tasks. The following are some of the exercises a patient's OT may do with him.

Everyday Chores

Depending on his abilities, a stroke survivor will work on brushing his teeth, washing his face, shaving, taking a shower, washing his hair, brushing his hair, and putting on clean clothes. These activities will likely leave him exhausted at first, but gradually his stamina will improve. They will eventually make him feel relaxed, fresh, and one step closer to being independent again.

He may also be placed in a practice kitchen to work on opening drawers, putting things on shelves, and moving things from the cabinet to the counter. He may practice opening a can of soup, pouring it into a pan, heating it up on the stove (taking care not to spill any or burn himself), and safely pouring the soup into a bowl. He may practice eating, cutting up his food with a knife, bringing his spoon or fork to his mouth, chewing and swallowing, and lifting up his glass to his mouth to drink. All these tasks require fine motor skills and coordination, and may seem difficult and annoying, as they were once simple tasks done with ease just a short time ago.

Another activity he may practice is washing his clothes in a washer and dryer. In the rehabilitation unit, he will be wearing his usual daily clothes, so he will need to wash these items from time to time. Eventually, he may be able to take his clothes, put them in the washer, pour in detergent, set the dial, and come back when they are done. Then he will put them in a dryer and set the dial. After the clothes are dry, he will remove them and fold them into piles and take them back to his room to put away. He may not be able to do all these tasks at first—maybe he will only be capable of folding his clean clothes at the beginning. That's fine; it's progress. He should enjoy each step forward and give himself a pat on the back.

Reaction Time and Rhythmic Exercises

There are numerous activities to improve reaction time. A patient may practice rhythmic activities to help his brain reestablish connections between nerve cells that have been damaged. A metronome can be used to keep the beat, or there are websites and apps available to help a stroke patient practice his reaction time. (See page 288 of the Resources.) He may find enjoyment in using these tools as he watches his reaction time improve.

Another option for doing rhythmic exercises is for a patient to listen to music and move—even if it's just fingers or toes—to the rhythm of his favorite songs, especially those with a distinctive beat, and even clap along, provided he doesn't have a roommate. Doing so can help heal brain damage and bring a little pleasure and relaxation into a stroke survivor's life.

Keyboarding Activities

If a patient routinely typed prior to the stroke, his OT may be able to provide him with a keyboard or laptop to practice, or a family member could bring a laptop from home. An OT will give a patient suggestions on how to relearn this skill if he is struggling. In addition, there are technological resources available to help a person regain typing skills or address difficulties, such as an adapted mouse or keypad, or voice-to-text software. Keyboarding isn't easy, as it requires combining very fine motor skills in both hands and all fingers while also relying on visual skills, concentration, and memory. A stroke survivor should not be surprised or discouraged if his first effort is gibberish. There are also websites that can be used to evaluate and practice typing. (See page 288 of the Resources.) He should not be too hard on himself if he seems to be hitting lots of incorrect keys. As he practices, more and more links between brain cells and the action of his hands will be created. Time, practice, and patience will help him improve greatly.

Using Tools

If a stroke survivor's occupation involves the use of tools, his OT will have similar items with which he can practice, such as nuts and bolts, screwdrivers, or pliers. The rehabilitation facility may even have a small workshop for patients to use. Using tools requires fine motor skills, coordination, and cognitive planning. For example, using pliers involves the use of small muscle coordination and strength in the hand, wrist, and lower and upper arms. Using a screwdriver also involves fine motor coordination and the ability to use one hand to hold the screwdriver and the other to hold the screw in place. These are not easy skills, so patience is an important quality for a person in rehabilitation to have. After all, some people struggle with these tasks even if they haven't had a stroke!

OT Equipment

The following pieces of equipment may be found in many rehabilitation facilities for occupational therapy:

- Bedside commode and shower chair
- Bed, dresser, sofa, and recliner chair
- Stove, dishwasher, washing machine, and dryer
- Dishes and silverware
- Peg boards, small blocks, and other small objects for fine motor exercise
- Mat, table, and yoga ball
- Large boards with lights to practice reaction time (e.g., whack-a-mole, Dynavision)
- Hand dynamometer (measures grip strength)

- Brake and accelerator pedals
- Sound equipment to practice reaction time
- Gaming equipment (e.g., Nintendo, Playstation)
- Electrical stimulation and robotic devices (e.g., Bioness, Hand Mentor)

OCCUPATIONAL OUTPATIENT THERAPY

Once a stroke survivor has left the hospital or acute rehabilitation unit, his OT will continue. His new therapist will want to know how things are going, how he is coping, and which activities are posing the most difficulty in order to design a program tailored to fit his needs. It may be difficult to for him to go to his medical and therapy appointments because he will not be driving yet. (See page 259 for ways to address this problem.) Nevertheless, going to therapy is extremely important for accelerating recovery. He should try not to miss any sessions. If he is also receiving other types of therapy, he may want to schedule these appointments back-to-back on the same day. If he is unable to go to his therapist, his therapist may be able to come to him or suggest websites that can guide him during at-home exercise. (See page 289 of the Resources.)

He may be exhausted when he gets home from outpatient therapy, so he should rest. This fatigue may be discouraging at first but will improve as he gets better. He should not schedule other major activities that sap him of energy on therapy days.

Advice for Caregivers
OCCUPATIONAL THERAPY AT HOME

Rehabilitation exercises don't end in the hospital, rehabilitation unit, or outpatient therapy. You should encourage a loved one who has experienced a stroke to continue his exercises at home. Help him settle into a routine at home that includes time for therapy. His daily routine will be a form of therapy in itself—getting bathed, brushing his teeth, buttoning his shirt or slipping it on over his head, and tying his shoes. Here are some ways you could help your loved one work on his recovery at home:

- If one of his hands is paralyzed or weak, help him use the other hand to bend his weak hand back towards his wrist and then down to his wrist. If he is able, he should do each hand by itself.

- Ask him to face his palm up and bring his thumb to his pinky finger, first to the base and then to the tip. Then he should touch his thumb to each finger in turn.

- Put pocket change, poker chips, or buttons in a cup and have him practice putting one item at a time into another cup. He should do this activity with each hand but concentrate on his weaker one.

- If his coordination is progressing, ask him to try to play the itsy-bitsy spider! (Perhaps his grandchildren could do it with him.) The best part of the itsy-bitsy spider is that it requires both hands, so that both sides of the brain must work together. It also uses many hand and finger muscles.

- Ask him to stack coins, poker chips, or small blocks with both hands.

- Help him put together an easy jigsaw puzzle of no more than thirty pieces. To do this he'll need to use his brain to figure out how to get started, how to turn over the puzzle pieces, how to put pieces of one color together, and how to fit the outside pieces together. This will require multiple brain processes, interpreting visual signals and coordinating his fingers all at the same time. He will feel proud of his finished puzzle. Next, try a puzzle with more pieces.

- Ask him to pick up five to ten dry beans and hold them in his hand. Then, from that hand, ask him to put the beans one by one in a cup. This is not as easy as it sounds, but with practice he'll get better.

- Ask him to practice squeezing a soft ball, such as a Nerf ball, as hard as he can.

- Ask him to roll a soft ball along a flat surface.

- Suggest he use child-sized building blocks that snap together to make simple structures. As his coordination improves, he can build bigger and more complicated structures. This activity will test the ability of his brain and hands to work together.

These can be fun activities, but if your loved one seems frustrated while doing them, don't push him too hard. There are enough other exercises that may be less discouraging for him to do.

CONCLUSION

Now that you understand the concept of occupational therapy—what OT is, how it can help stroke survivors, and the tests and tasks that a stroke patient may be required to perform in an intensive care unit, in rehab, or at home—it is time to learn about physical therapy, which is meant to help stroke survivors regain physical function, mobility, and balance. Like OT, PT can be incredibly challenging and may make a stroke survivor tired, but it will most likely improve his abilities to do everyday things and live independently.

6

Physical Therapy

While occupational therapy is designed to help a patient regain his ability to perform normal everyday activities, physical therapy, or PT (which may also be used to refer to a physical therapist), aims to improve a patient's capacity for general physical movement of his body. Physical therapy, sometimes called physiotherapy, uses special exercises and devices to restore physical function to the large muscles after a stroke. If a stroke patient has problems with limb movement, standing, walking, or balance, physical therapy will be helpful.

Like occupational therapists, physical therapists are highly educated and experienced professionals. They must have at least a master's degree in PT, complete an internship, and possess a state license. If you have ever broken a leg or arm, or had a knee replaced, you have probably seen a physical therapist. Physical therapy helps people live more actively after a stroke, illness, injury, or disability. While OT focuses on routine life tasks, PT addresses overall mobility.

A stroke survivor must work on improving his balance and regaining his coordination and strength in order to improve his mobility. Physical therapists test these abilities and develop exercise plans to improve them. After a person has a stroke, he may feel wobbly or unsteady when standing. He may even feel lightheaded while sitting on his bed or in a chair. These feelings will improve with time. In the meantime, his PT will put a belt around his waist to keep him from falling during exercises. The most improvement often occurs in the first few weeks after a stroke, but balance can improve slowly over months or even years, so he should try to persevere.

Weakness is a common problem for many stroke survivors, which limits their mobility. A physical therapist will start by working on transfers, such as from bed to wheelchair, or from wheelchair to toilet. She will also determine which device would likely be best for enhancing mobility, whether it is a wheelchair, walker, cane, or orthosis (brace). Whichever is right for a patient at the outset may be changed later as strength improves.

A physical therapist works with a patient to devise an at-home exercise program and may even teach his family or caregivers how to help. Of course, the specific set of exercises will depend on the patient's strength, balance, and coordination. The process may be frustrating, so the care team, family, and caregivers will need to provide encouragement to work hard on these skills, which are crucial to the achievement of any other goals he may set.

SETTING GOALS

Before specific goals can be determined, there are important factors to consider. Based on the severity of a patient's stroke, a PT will speak to either the patient or the patient's loved ones or caregivers to set realistic, meaningful goals for the patient.

Living Arrangements

A patient's therapy team will speak to him about his living environment. The timing of his return home will depend on numerous factors, including how much help he will need, who will be available to help him, how his house is set up, and the severity of any weakness, numbness, balance problems, or coordination problems he may be experiencing. The team will then set goals with the patient. If his long-term goal is to return to home, he may have several short-term goals, such as being able to move himself around in his wheelchair. He will need to work on standing up from a sitting position so he can get out of a chair or bed, transferring to a wheelchair, and standing up from a wheelchair to get back into bed. If he is going to use a cane, he will need to practice with it until he can move around various objects without stumbling. If he has stairs, he may wish to practice going up and down stairs in the PT room. Often, a PT will go to a patient's house to see the challenges he will need to overcome.

Daily Activities

A stroke patient's PT will want to know how he lived before the stroke. Did he prepare his own meals? While his OT will address this activity specifically, related elements such as strength and the ability to stand and balance will be the territory of his PT.

Physical therapy will work on the balance required to carry out daily personal care activities, which include brushing teeth, shaving, combing hair, showering, sitting on a toilet, and standing up from a toilet. Physical and occupational therapists will ask a lot of questions about a patient's house. For example, does he have grips in his bathtub so he does not slip? If not, does he have someone who could install these for him? Are there any tripping hazards present, such as mats?

Will he eventually be able to do his own grocery shopping? A shopping cart can help him keep his balance (most stores have riding carts he could use if fatigue or weakness is a problem). Balance will also be a factor in his taking a box from a high shelf and putting it in his cart. Of course, he will need both strength and balance to transfer his groceries from his shopping cart to his car.

Work Skills

If a patient is planning to return to work, physical therapy can help. A physical therapist will ask what kinds of physical abilities a patient will need to have in order to work. Will he need to walk up and down stairs? How far will he have to walk to his work area? How will he get to work? What physical skills are required for him to do his job? Can he go back to work part-time? Can he work from home on some days?

Leisure Activities

A patient's PT will want to know what leisure activities he enjoyed before his stroke. Did he play any sports? Is one of his goals to be able to engage in sports again? What physical abilities will he need to do so? For example, if he was a golfer, he and his PT could discuss whether golfing might be a reasonable goal. (With golf carts, he wouldn't need to be able to walk the course.) Is he ready to start swinging his golf club or do a little putting in a PT environment? If he enjoyed tennis, is he ready to grab a racket and hit some balloons or perhaps even a tennis ball against a wall? If he is able to accomplish these easy golf or tennis skills, his confidence will soar, and he will feel happier, more optimistic, and more motivated to accomplish other goals.

If he was a runner and wants to return to jogging, he could make that a long-term goal. He will need to work on balance, walking, and strengthening his legs. Gradually, during therapy, he can increase the distance and perhaps the pace of his walking as he gets stronger and steadier on his feet.

As goals are discussed, there are a number of important considerations to keep in mind. Are the goals realistic—both physically and financially? Will he have a network of family members and friends to rely on? Is his living arrangement adequate enough given his limitations? Is he psychologically prepared to meet the challenges that lie ahead of him?

Advice for Caregivers
ATTENDING PT SESSIONS

As with OT, you should try to go to your loved one's PT sessions, where you can encourage him, observe his weaknesses, see the types of exercises he is working on, and ask questions. Ask his therapist if there are any exercises he could do in his room. Of course, when he leaves rehabilitation, his PT will give him exercises to do at home.

PHYSICAL THERAPY EVALUATION

As you learned in Chapter 1, the effects of a stroke can vary in severity, ranging from mild to severe. The following are stroke-related issues that a PT will evaluate and help a stroke survivor correct or greatly improve:

- **Weakness.** This issue is typically due to paralysis of muscles on one side of the body. For example, a patient's left face, arm, and leg may have been affected by a stroke that occurred on the right side of his brain.

- **Uncoordinated Movement.** This issue refers to when a patient's leg or arm on the affected side does not respond to movement orders from his brain. His hip may move up when he wants it to move forward.

- **Abnormal Sensations.** This issue refers to feelings of numbness, pins and needles, or pain on one side of the body, or even to an inability to feel pain or temperature.

- **Inability to Sit or Stand Straight.** This issue refers to balance and posture problems, which could lead to falls.

- **Muscle Inflexibility.** This issue refers to stiffness in muscles in the arms and legs, which makes it difficult for a patient to move.

- **Muscle Spasms.** Muscle spasms refer to when muscles contract suddenly and sometimes painfully.

Physical Therapy Tests

A physical therapist will do various tests to determine a stroke patient's strength and balance. These tests help a PT set goals with a patient, ensuring that both short- and long-term goals are realistic and achievable.

Strength Tests

Muscle weakness is common after stroke. A physical therapist will test how well a patient can move in his bed—can he roll over, move his legs and arms, or even sit up in bed? His doctor, nurse, and PT will decide if he is able to sit in a chair. The more he moves, the more he will be able to move.

A PT will evaluate a patient's strength by testing each muscle group. In doing so, she may ask him to lift his arm while she pushes down on it, bend his arm at the elbow, straighten his arm and hold his hand like he is stopping traffic, or open his fingers. She will compare the strength of his affected side with that of his unaffected side. She may ask him to squeeze her fingers as hard as he can. She may test—even measure with an instrument—to see how far he can move his head—up and down, and side to side. Periodically, she will re-test him to make sure he is improving, sharing the results with him. If he has not improved she may try other exercises to accomplish the same goals.

Balance Tests

A physical therapist will want to know if a stroke patient feels unsteady, dizzy, or lightheaded when he sits up in bed or stands. Does he feel like he is spinning? Does it seem as though the world around him is spinning? Does he feel like he may faint?

Did you know that your sense of balance depends on your ears, eyes, balance center in the brain (cerebellum), and nerves in your feet all working together with your brain? For this reason, a physical therapist will check a patient's sensation and vision. At some point, she may put a strap around his waist so she can hold on to him—whether he weighs 100 pounds or 300 pounds. If his balance problems are severe, his therapist may refer him to another PT who has had special training in balance therapy, also called vestibular therapy.

PHYSICAL THERAPY EXERCISES AND ACTIVITIES

After evaluating a patient, a physical therapist will develop a treatment plan. Like all forms of therapy, repetition is the key. A patient will do his exercises, rest, do them again, rest, and so on.

Strength

Based on his test results, a stroke patient's PT will provide exercises aimed at improving his strength. The more he does these exercises, the sooner his strength will return. His stamina—the ability to exercise without fatigue—will also benefit. She may also suggest gentle stretching exercises if his muscles and joints are stiff. These movements may be hard work, resulting in exhaustion. This outcome is perfectly normal.

Balance

A stroke patient can help his recovery simply by getting moving after having had a stroke. Thankfully, physical therapy typically starts as soon as a patient is stable in the ICU or recovery ward. A physical therapist will help a patient sit up in bed, sit on the edge of the bed, and eventually stand next to the bed. A patient will need someone to bring good walking shoes for him to wear, or his rehabilitation unit may provide special socks that grip the floor to prevent him from slipping. He should wear his glasses if he normally wears glasses, and also wear his hearing aid if he has one.

In the PT room, he may do all kinds of activities to improve balance. He may practice standing while holding on to a rail and then without a rail. He may practice standing on one foot and then on the other while holding on to a rail and then without a rail. He may stand on a soft mat to practice standing on a floor that is not quite firm, first with his eyes open and then with them closed. His eyes aid in balance, so staying steady will be a challenge without visual input. It's a little like practicing standing on one foot. In normal life, he won't be standing on just one foot—or keeping his eyes closed—but these exercises will improve his ability to balance.

Gait

Gait refers to a person's manner of walking. If a patient can stand and balance reasonably well, he could try to take a step with the support of a walker. He may try to move his legs while holding on to parallel bars. It may be difficult at first to take that first step, but his therapist will help him, and the more steps he takes, the better he will get at walking. His brain and legs will need to re-learn how to work together, so he should be patient with himself. He should feel proud and happy after taking those first few steps and realize he is actually moving on his own. At some point, he may move to using a cane as a walking aid. Finally, he may try to take a few steps without the help of a walker or cane. Doing so will be reason enough for a victory party, but after that he will need to practice his walking again and again until he can move around the therapy room and finally back to his room—always with his therapist attached to him by a belt.

If he is doing well, his physical therapist may put him on a treadmill at a slow speed. (If balance is an issue, she may have him use a harness.) This exercise will help improve the rhythm of his gait. Even if his balance and walking have improved, his physical therapist may still recommend the use of a walker or cane when he goes home—at least at first.

Spasticity

As you learned in Chapter 4, after a stroke, a survivor's affected side may develop spasticity, which refers to continuous muscle contractions that can by painful. Spasticity can result in tight fists, bent elbows, or stiff arms, fingers, legs, and knees. Physical therapists and physicians have ways to reduce spasticity.

A physical therapist may put a brace on an affected muscle and joint, help with range-of-motion exercises, or gently stretch affected muscles. She may use *functional electrical stimulation* (FES) to treat a painful or stiff joint. A physician may prescribe medications to help a patient with spasticity, give him injections that block the chemicals that make his muscles tight, or even recommend surgery to block the pain and restore normal movement. Thankfully, his doctor and PT will have many different methods to relieve pain and stiffness.

PT Equipment

Just as occupational therapy has its own specialized equipment, the following equipment may be found in many rehabilitation facilities for PT:

- Large balls
- Bumpy pads to walk on to improve balance
- Large boxes with sides that move and a floor that can tip to measure and improve balance
- Parallel bars to help with walking
- Bar to treat and improve balance
- Treadmill

OUTPATIENT PHYSICAL THERAPY

Once a stroke patient has returned home or is in a short- or long-term facility, his therapy will likely continue with a different therapist. He may do similar activities to those he did in rehabilitation. The key to improvement is practice, practice, and more practice. His new PT will want to know how things are going—has he had any falls and, if so, under what circumstances? Is he in any pain and, if so, has he called the doctor? Has he been able to increase the distance he moves using a wheelchair, walker, or cane, or on his own? She will ask about his balance—does he feel steady? Is his weakness improving? What does he think he needs to improve?

Outpatient PT can be tiring, but gradually stamina and strength improve. After PT, he should rest without sleeping. Sleeping or napping during the day can alter the sleep-wake cycle, causing insomnia or poor sleep at night.

Physical Therapy at Home

A stroke survivor's therapist will likely give him exercises to do at home. A friend, loved one, or caregiver can help him make a daily schedule that includes PT and other therapeutic exercises. He may want to do physical therapy in the morning and occupational therapy in the afternoon. Simply living—moving around the home, going up and down stairs, helping to fix a healthy meal—will be therapeutic, too.

The following exercises may form part of a stroke patient's at-home therapy, but no stroke survivor should attempt any of these movements without the approval of his physical therapist. Treatment can vary so much between stroke survivors, so a PT must evaluate a patient before recommending at-home exercises. Safety is crucial. After all, a patient won't have his therapist holding on to his belt to keep him from falling during at-home physical therapy.

Wheelchair Exercises

Just because a stroke survivor is in a wheelchair does not mean he cannot engage in a number of exercises that can improve his strength and coordination. A PT may recommend lifting light weights and increasing repetitions according to ability. She may suggest playing catch with a loved one (using a Nerf ball or a larger ball). A patient may also practice bending and straightening the knee of his weak leg over and over again. Then he could try the same movement with his unaffected leg. A patient may be told to try raising both arms as high as possible, clapping, and then bringing his arms back to his sides. If his neighborhood is safe, he may want to wheel himself around outside in his wheelchair, gradually increasing his distance. Getting out in the sun will feel wonderful and the sunlight will allow his body to produce vitamin D.

Standing and Walking Exercises

As an at-home exercise, if a stroke survivor is able to stand, his therapist may tell him to hold on to the back of a chair and then remain standing for a few seconds without holding it. Always ready to grab the chair again if necessary, he could then try to increase the time spent not holding the back of the chair. While holding on to the back of the chair, he could try lifting one foot for a few seconds and then do the same with the other foot. If he is quite stable, he could try this exercise without holding on to the chair, gradually increasing the time spent with one foot lifted. Holding on to the back of the chair, he could try putting one foot directly in front of the other (with the heel of one touching the toe of the other). He could also try the same exercise without holding on to the chair. If it goes well, with his PT's permission, he might use this method to try walking.

If a patient has a stationary bike, he may use it at home, biking for ten seconds, resting, and then repeating. He may try to increase this time until he is able to bike for ten minutes, or even twenty minutes. Doing so will help him rebuild his strength, stamina, and coordination, and reduce his risk of having another stroke.

For a stroke patient, simply walking around the house can benefit recovery. He may also listen to music that has a very definite rhythm and try to dance to it. If he is in a wheelchair, he could clap to the beat. Practicing his walking skills outdoors may provide a welcome change from his usual surroundings, offering fresh air and sunlight. Of course, a patient should never try any of these at-home exercises without first attaining approval from his physical therapist.

CONCLUSION

By working to rebuild balance, strength, and mobility, physical therapy plays a crucial role in a stroke patient's recovery. These elements are necessary for a survivor to regain as much of his old life as possible. A patient requires proper balance, strength, and mobility in order to perform the exercises he needs to do to see progress in his rehabilitation. And when it comes to physical therapy, the earlier it is undertaken, the better. Stroke patients should get moving as soon as possible, and move as often as possible, but never without the guidance of a physical therapist.

7

$\int$ peech Therapy

While occupational therapy and physical therapy help stroke survivors improve their mobility and capacity for everyday tasks, speech therapy helps them manage any swallowing, communication, or cognitive problems, which often remain after a stroke. Approximately half of all stroke survivors have difficulty swallowing after stroke. About one in three stroke survivors has difficulties in communicating (i.e., speaking, understanding, reading, or writing). In fact, as you learned in Chapter 1, speech difficulties are typically one of the first symptoms of a stroke and an indication that someone needs to call 911 immediately. About one in five stroke survivors also develops memory problems in the first three months, and at five years, one in three have memory difficulties.

A speech therapist, or ST (which may also be used to refer to speech therapy), plays just as important a role in a stroke patient's rehabilitation as an occupational therapist or physical therapist. A speech therapist is highly educated—typically having a master's degree, an internship, and certification—to assess and treat communication problems, thinking problems, and swallowing problems, which are often due to a neurological condition.

DIFFICULTY SWALLOWING

Swallowing is something we all take for granted, but a stroke survivor's ability to swallow after a stroke may be impaired. Difficulty swallowing, known as dysphagia, is a problem that affects about half of all stroke patients. Just as the muscles of a patient's arm or leg can be paralyzed or weakened by a stroke, so can the muscles of a patient's throat or tongue.

People with dysphagia may have difficulty drinking, eating, swallowing pills, or controlling saliva. These problems may be obvious or observable only through specialized examinations (i.e., silent dysphagia). Problems associated with dysphagia may include coughing or choking when eating or drinking, which can lead to liquid or food going down the wrong pipe and ending up in the lungs, known as aspiration. This problem can cause a serious, life-threatening lung infection known as pneumonia. Other patients with dysphagia may have sensory deficits as well as muscular deficits, which can make them unaware of problems with the swallowing process and put them at risk of aspiration. An inability to swallow food properly may lead to malnutrition or dehydration. Thankfully, speech therapists are trained to address this issue.

A stroke survivor may meet his speech therapist in the emergency department, intensive care unit, or hospital ward soon after his stroke, as it is critical to assess his ability to swallow before he is given anything to drink or eat. As soon as a stroke patient has been stabilized, his speech therapist will test his swallowing. She will watch to see how he chews and swallows, and how well the muscles in his mouth and throat work. She may ask his doctor to order an x-ray to determine how the swallowing process has been affected, and which exercises or eating modifications might make eating safer for him. This evaluation will indicate whether foods and liquids of different consistencies are going into the lungs instead of the stomach, which would put the patient at risk of acquiring pneumonia. If problems are observed, his speech therapist will provide exercises and suggest other strategies to make swallowing safer for him.

If a patient has mild swallowing problems, it may be necessary to alter the texture of certain foods so he can swallow them. Thick drinks and smooth puréed foods will go down easier than thin beverages—like water—or regular food. If he has severe problems, a feeding tube may be inserted through his nose, down his throat, and into his stomach so he receives adequate nutrition. If his swallowing problems persist, his doctor may choose to insert a tube from outside his abdomen, through his skin and muscle, into his stomach.

A stroke survivor's speech therapist will work with his nurse, doctor, dietitian, and other team members to come up with a plan organized just for him. If he is able to eat or drink, she may advise him to take only small sips of thickened fluids, as thin fluids may be riskier to swallow. She will recommend that he sit up straight anytime he is drinking or eating. She may tell him to turn his head to one side while eating or drinking, which may help protect his airway.

A stroke patient should not be rushed when eating. He should be allowed to chew his food well and make sure it all leaves his mouth on its trip to his stomach. His speech therapist will recommend which foods and beverages he can manage and which must be modified. A patient's swallowing therapy exercise program may include heat or electrical stimulation therapy to improve the sensory feedback and movement involved in swallowing. Therapists typically welcome the involvement of caregivers in practicing these exercises with stroke survivors.

Advice for Caregivers
HELPING YOUR LOVED ONE WITH SWALLOWING

Observing your loved one with his speech therapist will be helpful. You will need to know what foods and drinks to avoid and exactly how to modify them for easier swallowing. His speech therapist will give you directions for preparing his food and beverages before he leaves the hospital. You will also learn the facial, tongue, and mouth exercises he will need to do each day. If his swallowing gets worse, you will need to let his doctor and speech therapist know immediately.

DIFFICULTY COMMUNICATING

In everyday vocabulary, the terms speech and language are often used interchangeably. Technically, however, speech refers to the physical and muscular aspect of producing sounds (including breathing, voicing, and articulating), while language refers to the symbolic system that is expressed in speech (including word meanings, sentence structure, and grammar). When a stroke affects a person's ability to produce speech, the disorder is termed *dysarthria*. A patient with dysarthria typically has slurred speech, which may be difficult to understand. When a stroke affects a person's ability to understand or formulate language, the disorder is called *aphasia*. Dysarthria and aphasia can occur together. During an evaluation, a speech therapist will determine whether the communication problems a stroke survivor is experiencing are primarily caused by speech, language, or cognitive factors (or a combination), and then design a therapy program accordingly.

It's important to understand that communication difficulties may linger after a stroke. These difficulties often improve with time but starting speech therapy as soon as possible is important. Whether the problem is a slight case of difficulty getting the words out or a full inability to speak or understand, a speech therapist will work with a stroke patient to help him regain the ability to communicate.

Forms of Aphasia

There are several types of aphasia, depending on which part of the brain is affected. Much depends upon the location of a patient's stroke and the patient's handedness. As mentioned earlier, in individuals who are right-handed, the speech centers are on the left side of the brain. Half of left-handed individuals have language function on the left and the other half have the language on the right. These areas are connected by networks of cells; therefore, interruption of these connections can cause difficulties speaking, understanding, repeating, and naming.

Depending on the type and severity of a stroke, a survivor may improve quickly or take many months or years to show improvements in the ability to communicate, so it is crucial for a patient not to give up on this goal too soon. In severe cases, aphasia is a chronic condition which survivors continue to live with and manage for the rest of their lives.

In order to understand the types of communication difficulties one can have after a stroke, it helps to know a little about certain types of aphasia.

Anomic Aphasia

Anomic aphasia, also called dysnomia, nominal aphasia, or amnesic aphasia, is a mild form of aphasia. While a patient is able to talk, he has problems retrieving or remembering words he would like to say. While he may know what he would like to say, he cannot connect it to the spoken word, especially when trying to use verbs and nouns.

Expressive (Broca's) Aphasia

In expressive aphasia, also known as Broca's aphasia, a patient can understand what is being said but has difficulty speaking or putting words together. His speech is often sparse, halting, and hesitant. Patients may make errors in which they use the wrong words or repeat words previously spoken. Given their preserved ability to understand, these patients often get frustrated by their difficulty communicating or mistakes. It is helpful to encourage them and to ask them "yes or no" questions.

Receptive (Wernicke's) Aphasia

Also called Wernicke's aphasia, receptive aphasia refers to the ability to speak words without understanding them. Given this lack of comprehension, a patient may be unaware that the words he is using are jumbled together. Such patients often do not get frustrated because they do not realize that what they are saying does not make sense. A patient with receptive aphasia is also unable to understand his own native language when it is spoken. What he hears instead sounds like an unfamiliar foreign language. Typically, patients with this type of aphasia are not able to communicate in writing either.

Global Aphasia

Global aphasia is a severe form of aphasia in which a patient is unable to understand or speak. Global aphasia is common early after the onset of stroke and can develop into other types of aphasia with time as a patient recovers the ability to speak or understand.

Mixed Transcortical Aphasia

Mixed transcortical aphasia is similar to global aphasia in that a patient is unable to communicate with or understand others. Mixed transcortical aphasia patients can, however, repeat words, phrases, or even long statements they hear without understanding what they are saying. In light of this form of aphasia, it is important to check a patient's ability to understand what he has said by asking follow-up questions.

Advice for Caregivers
UNDERSTANDING COMMUNICATION DIFFICULTIES

Most people have an idea of what a stroke can do to a person's mobility, but few of us understand the impact it can have on a person's ability to communicate with others. It's hard to imagine how difficult life can be without this ability until it is taken away. For a patient, it can feel incredibly frustrating. For family members, the shock of learning that a person they have spoken to every day and shared stories with is no longer able to communicate can be overwhelming. If you are a loved one of a stroke survivor, the more prepared you are to recognize the type of communication issues a stroke has brought on in his case, the better the position you will be in to talk to the person in charge of his speech rehabilitation.

Evaluation of Communication

A speech therapist will evaluate a patient's communication skills. She will test his speech, language, and comprehension using a number of techniques, including:

- **Spontaneous speech.** A speech therapist will engage in an introductory conversation with a patient. Later, she may ask him to describe pictures she shows to him. While the patient is speaking, she will assess the fluency of speech (ease of getting the words out) and speech content. Is the speech fluid without hesitation or halting and sparse? Does it make sense? Are there nonsensical words?

- **Repetition of words and sentences.** A speech therapist will ask a patient to repeat simple words or short sentences.

- **Comprehension.** A speech therapist will want to know if a patient can understand her when she asks him to show her two fingers, identify his nose, or point to the ceiling. She may also use "yes or no" questions, such as, "Is the lady next to you your wife?" or, "Is the sky green?"

Advice for Caregivers
PATIENCE AND COMMUNICATION PROBLEMS

As the saying goes, "Patience is a virtue." You will certainly need patience if a loved one is having communication problems after a stroke. He may have difficulty with his speech such that you cannot understand him, which will be frustrating for both of you. He may not understand your words, or he may be unable to read and write. Imagine what it must be like to wake up in a world in which everyone is speaking in a "foreign" language you don't understand. Or your loved one may know exactly what he wants to say but everything comes out as gibberish. He would have good reason to be terrified, extremely frustrated, or lonely. He may feel like a wall has been built between him and others, and that he is alone in his own little world.

Not surprisingly, your loved one may become very angry at you and the staff because you don't understand what he is trying to say. Try to assure him that you know he is trying very hard and that his speech will improve steadily if he works with his speech therapist. Be compassionate, positive, and respectful. Provide him with pictures of common objects to which he could point as an aid in his efforts to communicate, or see if he can draw pictures to show you. Try to keep the room quiet (no TV) during his speech exercises.

Here's where patience comes in. Speaking loudly or shouting won't help. Finishing his sentences for him will not help. Instead, give him plenty of time to find the words he is looking for so he can speak for himself. Speak simply, clearly, and slowly. If you don't understand what he is trying to say, don't pretend you do. Ask him politely to try again. Don't speak to him as though he were a child. Look him in the eye, smile, hold his hand, and be patient. Think of how you would feel if roles were reversed and you had communication problems.

- **The name game.** A speech therapist will want to know if a patient can name certain items. She may point to objects in the room or pictures of objects and ask him to name them.

- **Reading and writing.** A speech therapist may ask a patient to read a word, phrase, or short paragraph, and to write his name and maybe even his address. These reading and writing tests may not be part of the first testing session but will be included in a later evaluation.

SPEECH AND LANGUAGE THERAPY

Like other forms of stroke therapy, speech and language therapy, often simply called speech therapy, sets goals for a patient with input from his recovery team, loved ones, and the patient himself. The aim should be to recover as much of his speech as possible or to find other ways to communicate. His personal goals will depend on his age, whether he will be living alone, and whether he will be returning to work. Did he have vision or hearing problems before the stroke? If so, how are these problems since his stroke? Does he have memory problems? If he wears dentures, do they fit properly? All these factors will affect his ability to communicate.

The types of speech and language therapy his speech therapist recommends will depend on the speech and language problems he is having—there is no one size fits all. And just as with occupational therapy and physical therapy, repetition is the key to success in speech therapy. He will have to repeat, repeat, and repeat his tasks to recover his speech. A patient's speech therapist may also have handouts of pictures and words with which he can practice after therapy. Practice uses the brain's ability to rewire itself and work around a damaged area (i.e., neuroplasticity, as described in Chapter 1).

In the short term, there are apps a stroke survivor can use to send helpful messages to others (e.g., "I have communication problems and am unable to talk to you myself, but I can understand what you say"). To work on a stroke survivor's long-term speech and language recovery, a speech therapist may choose one or more of the following methods of therapy.

Repetition

A speech therapist may give a patient a word to repeat, starting, perhaps, with his name or the name of a family member. She may say simple sounds such as "ah, "oo," or "ee" and ask him to copy these sounds. Repetition of this exercise will help his ability to say targeted sounds and words. It may be frustrating, but repetition is important to establish new or strengthen old wiring in the brain's speech center after it has been damaged by a stroke.

A patient's speech therapist may ask him to repeat rhyming words, such as "bell, cell, fell, tell, well," or "sat, pat, hat, cat," and so on. She will start with short words and then move on to longer ones. She may ask him to repeat important short words such as "hi, bye, yes, no, up, down." She may ask him to say a short word like "pan" or "tooth" and then ask him to make it a longer word such as "pancake" or "toothache."

Visual Communication Therapy

A speech therapist may use index cards with words, symbols, or pictures on them to stimulate a patient's speech. She may ask him to point at pictures of different things—ball, baby, card, bed, dog, and so on. She may ask him to sort pictures of fruits and vegetables according to these categories. She may show him two words and him if they have the same meaning—for example, men and women, cats and dogs, dogs and puppies, pants and slacks, and so on.

Drawings

If a stroke patient is having problems speaking, his speech therapist may suggest he draw pictures of what he would like to communicate. He doesn't have to have artistic talent to do this—stick figures will be just fine. For example, he could draw a picture of a cup if he is thirsty, food if he is hungry, happy or sad faces to show his emotional state, or a toilet if he needs to use the bathroom. If he happens to have artistic talent, he may be able to express himself more completely in his art work, which may reduce his stress. The hospital may also have a communication board with pictures of common useful things to which a patient may point in order to communicate.

Words Put to Music

Typically, music is stored in a different part of the brain than speech. A speech therapist can take advantage of these neural pathways to produce speech. She may find a patient has an easier time singing the lyrics of short tunes rather than simply speaking the same words without the benefit of a tune. In other words, singing, "Row, Row, Row Your Boat," "Baa, Baa, Black Sheep," or the "ABC Song" may actually be useful. This exercise is not intended to treat a patient like a child but rather to stimulate the language center of his brain. As he masters simple songs, his speech therapist may choose more complicated, adult songs for him to sing, or perhaps he will come up with one or more songs on his own.

Even saying words in a sing-song or melodic manner may help. For example, saying "good morning" in a bright cheerful way almost has a melody. A speech therapist can encourage this kind of exaggerated speech for everyday communication to help a patient recover. Research has also shown that patients who listen to their favorite music become less confused or depressed. Just as important, it can help them recover mental function.

Gestures

A speech therapist will help a patient communicate in ways other than speech. For example, she may show him hand gestures he can use, such as pointing to objects or making the gesture of drinking something. This non-verbal communication may become a simplified sign language. A speech therapist can work with a patient to create signs for statements such as, "I love you," "I need a hug," and "I'm so depressed," or questions such as, "What time is it?" and so on. This non-verbal communication will help him connect with the outside world and strengthen new wiring in his brain.

SCIENTIFIC EVIDENCE FOR SPEECH THERAPY

A review of studies on aphasia found that speech therapy improved functional use of language, language comprehension (i.e., comprehension of written and spoken language), and language production (i.e., production of language through speech and the written word) when compared to no access to therapy, but it was unclear how long these benefits lasted. Although many studies have compared different types of speech therapy, which approach is best is still unclear. Short sessions of highly intensive therapy seem to work better than long sessions of less intensive therapy. Many hours of therapy over a short term (e.g., ten hours a week for three weeks) appear to help patients' language use in daily life and reduce the severity of their aphasia problems.

At-Home Speech Therapy

There are many speech therapy exercises that can be done at home. A speech therapist may ask a patient's loved ones to do the following at home with him:

- Take out his family picture album and ask him to say who the people are and where the pictures were taken.

- Assemble his old photos and organize them into an album. Perhaps he can help you write a caption for each picture.

- Look at the daily newspaper and discuss the date and day of the week. Talk about the time. If he wore a watch before his stroke, make sure he still wears it. Get him a watch that gives the date and day of the week if his current watch does not. Read a newspaper story to him or ask him to read it. Look at the comics section and have one of you read the words.

- Try a very simple crossword puzzle together, helping him choose the right words and spellings. Look for very simple puzzles at your pharmacy, grocery store, bookstore, or online.

- Talk about the weather and all the words to describe it—rain, snow, thunder, lightning, sunny, and so on. Buy a simple book that has many rhyming words, such as such as a Dr. Seuss book. Read it aloud or help him say the words and try to read some simple sentences. He may enjoy rhyming poems that have particular rhythms to them.

- Find objects in different colors, like paint samples, and identify primary colors—red, blue, yellow—and secondary colors—purple, green, orange. Include black and white as well. Play a guessing game of "I see something that is blue and large (the carpet)" or "I see something that is white and fluffy (the cat)."

- Play his favorite music. Sing along with the lyrics. Encourage him to sing, too.

With any at-home speech therapy exercise, the goal is to increase a patient's vocabulary, strengthen his ability to say words and sentences, and perhaps improve his ability to write. Speech therapy sessions and at-home exercises should provide a stroke survivor with opportunities to express his thoughts on topics he finds meaningful. A patient's caregivers and family members can provide invaluable background information, if necessary, to help his therapist cater activities to his likes, which may motivate him to practice.

COGNITIVE IMPAIRMENT

Approximately one in five stroke survivors develop cognitive impairment after stroke. Cognitive impairment is a precursor to dementia. Risk factors for dementia after stroke include older age, lower education level, previous stroke, type 2 diabetes, atrial fibrillation, cognitive impairment prior to stroke, and higher stroke severity.

Cognition consists of several elements, including attention, concentration, memory, language, visuospatial skills (i.e., the ability to interpret the spatial relationships of objects in the visual field), calculation, and orientation (e.g., a person's knowledge of his location and the date).

Depending on how a stroke has affected the brain (areas and severity), cognitive problems may range from very mild to extremely disabling. A speech therapist will perform various tests according to a stroke survivor's individual situation. Initially, in order to determine if a patient is oriented, a speech therapist will ask him to say his name, the date, the place in which he is located, and the reason for his hospitalization. It is extremely rare for a person to forget his own identity, but some stroke survivors do experience confusion about dates, locations, and reasons for hospitalization. A speech therapist may also recommend additional neuropsychological testing by a specialized psychologist.

The most common tests used to test a stroke survivor's cognitive function are the Montreal Cognitive Assessment (MoCA) and the Mini Mental State Examination (MMSE). The MoCA asks patients to perform tasks such as drawing a clock and marking a certain time on it; connecting dots in sequence; identifying the names of the animals pictured; repeating a list of words; reading lists of digits (one list to be read forwards, a shorter list to be read backwards); subtracting numbers by a factor of seven; stating the date, month, year, and day; and identifying their current locations.

The MMSE includes questions on similar subject matter—naming objects, drawing a picture, counting backwards, identifying the date, etc.—and both assign a numerical score to each question or task. The total score of each test corresponds to a designated level of cognitive impairment.

Cognitive Rehabilitation

Cognitive rehabilitation typically focuses on reinforcing or reestablishing previous behavioral skills or functions and teaching compensatory strategies. A speech therapist will use different techniques to treat the various cognitive issues that may be present in a patient after he has experienced a stroke.

Orientation

For a patient who is disoriented, it is helpful for a therapist to explain gently and in simple terms what has happened to him, where he is, and what the date is. It will also be helpful for a patient to keep a calendar handy, and to write down and review each day's activities with his therapist. Hospital staff will frequently check whether a patient's disorientation is resolving as an indicator of his recovery pattern. Keep in mind that hospitals can be disorienting, particularly for older individuals. A patient's sleep-wake cycle is often disrupted in the hospital, with nurses checking his blood pressure and giving him medication in the middle of the night, bright light coming into his room from the hallway, roommates making noise, and, in some circumstances, no natural sunlight to be found. A patient may be able to get back on a less disorienting schedule by avoiding daytime naps, limiting visitors and phone calls at night, and keeping the lights on during the day and off at night.

Memory

Memory is typically understood as the recall of past events, but a stroke that causes memory problems tends to impair the brain's ability to form new memories, leaving memories made before the stroke intact. Therefore, a stroke survivor may not recall who came to visit him in the hospital yesterday while still being able to recall life experiences from childhood or several years prior. Since memory does not work like a tape recorder, equally preserving all experienced events and facts, family members may find it frustrating that a stroke survivor remembers some things and forgets others. Often, a stroke survivor is unaware of his memory problem and has difficulty using techniques to improve it.

A speech therapist will try out various techniques (using a calendar, writing lists, using cell phone reminders, etc.) to see which ones are helpful and easily adopted. If a survivor used certain organizational methods to remember things prior to his stroke, it is typically easier to retrain his memory by using this system than for him to learn via other techniques. Any insight that a patient's family can provide into his daily routine or other familiar memory strategies will help in the management of memory problems.

Neglect

A stroke that affects the right side of the brain may result in a survivor having problems processing sensory information that comes from the other side of the body, also known as *neglect*. It may seem as though a stroke patient is not seeing properly, and he may even say, "I need new glasses," but the problem may be caused by damage to the part of the brain that processes what he sees. Family members may observe him having trouble finding food on the left side of his plate, seeming to ignore people who are stand on his left side, or misreading words and sentences. All the therapists on his healthcare team will practice activities to address any problems with his visuospatial skills within their areas of focus.

When a person has a conversation with someone who has had a stroke, it may be better to first get his attention on his right side, where it is easiest for him to process information, and then gradually move to his left and see how successfully he can stay in the conversation as his visuospatial skills are increasingly challenged. He may give nonverbal signs that he is getting frustrated or fatigued before it becomes too difficult.

Problem-Solving, Insight, and Safety

Depending on the severity of cognitive problems a stroke survivor experiences, solving daily problems (e.g., finding a lost item, balancing a checking account or driving to an unfamiliar location) may become difficult or even impossible for him to manage without assistance. He may try to do things too impulsively without thinking through the possible consequences, or he may be able to see that something needs to be done but have difficulty starting and following through on actions (i.e., initiation problems).

Some stroke survivors have difficulty recognizing stroke-related physical or cognitive changes (i.e., lack of insight). These issues may exist in various combinations and be differently affected by personal factors (e.g., fatigue, lack of sleep) or environmental situations (e.g., unfamiliar places, loud noises). These concerns may put a stroke survivor's safety at risk. His speech therapist or other members of his rehabilitation team may recommend he be supervised to ensure his safety at home or during activities in the community. Observing a stroke survivor actually engaging in therapy will help family members better understand how much help he needs. There is often a gap between what a patient is able to talk about doing and what he is able to do.

Advice for Caregivers
DECISION-MAKING

If a loved one has had a stroke, you may find he is no longer able understand complicated issues such as finances. He may not be able to make important financial decisions or express his wishes about his healthcare. You will want to discuss your observations and concerns with his doctor, speech therapist, social worker, and close family members. These cognitive problems may be temporary or long term. To address immediate issues, you may need to obtain power of attorney, which is a legal document that allows an individual to appoint someone else as manager of his affairs, provided he is considered legally capable of making this decision. Power of attorney will be required in order for you to sign documents and make decisions about his healthcare on his behalf.

A patient may, however, have a living will that spells out his desires in matters of healthcare. A living will is a document that allows an individual to communicate his healthcare wishes in the event that he is unable to do so due to illness. If a stroke survivor has a living will, it should be added to his medical chart. You may need to speak to an attorney to set up any necessary legal documents when it comes to decision-making.

CONCLUSION

As is the case in occupational therapy and physical therapy, repetition is the key to making progress in speech therapy. Repetition of speech will help a stroke survivor's brain rewire itself, allowing him to communicate again. This process may be frustrating, but if he persists and follows the recommendations of his speech therapist, he can continue to improve. Recovery from aphasia and cognitive problems is typically slower than recovery from physical problems. Moreover, a patient may go through periods in which no progress in speech is evident, but each of these periods is likely to be followed by new gains eventually.

While traditional therapies such as occupational therapy, physical therapy, and speech therapy are the mainstay of stroke recovery, there are complementary therapies that may also be quite helpful to stroke survivors, as the next chapter discusses. Some of these therapies are even becoming part of the mainstream.

8

*C*omplementary
Therapies

Previous chapters of this book have discussed treatments that are traditionally given to a stroke patient in order to restore blood flow to the brain and minimize damage from a stroke. These therapies are known as "standard," "Western," or "mainstream" treatments. They have been studied extensively, commonly practiced for many years, and proven to work.

This chapter focuses on other therapies for stroke patients—nonstandard therapies about which you may not have heard, or about which you may have questions. These options may be considered *complementary medicine.* Complementary medicine is meant to be used alongside traditional treatment options. Some of these treatments have been used for thousands of years in Asia and some areas of Europe. Most complementary therapies are safe if provided by trained professionals. Although some of the therapies mentioned in this chapter may have undergone investigation by researchers, they have not been subject to as much rigorous study as have mainstream medical therapies.

Conducting research is complicated. The most rigorous type of clinical trial is a double-blind randomized controlled clinical trial. In this type of study, there are two groups with similar characteristics (e.g., age, gender, type of stroke, or race). Each person is randomly assigned to the trial's treatment group, which receives the medication being studied, or the trial's control group, which is given a *placebo*—a look-a-like tablet or capsule that is medically inactive. None of the participants are aware of which group they are in, nor do researchers check outcomes until a predetermined point in the study has been reached, at which time these outcomes are compared. Any side effects reported by the two groups are also compared.

This type of research may be difficult to perform in connection with some of the therapies discussed in this chapter. For example, there is no way to mask the scents of essential oils from a patient in a study of aromatherapy. In addition, research on yoga or tai chi can be done by comparing one group that performs the activity with a group that does not, but it is impossible for each group not to know the method of therapy it is testing.

Despite not being studied as much as mainstream therapies, many of these complementary treatments, including tai chi, yoga, music therapy, and aromatherapy, have entered the mainstream, and patients often have questions for their therapists about the use of these methods as recovery aids. This chapter is meant to address these questions.

The popularity of complementary therapies seems to grow every year. Currently it is estimated that far more Americans visit complementary therapists than their primary doctors each year, spending billions of dollars on complementary treatments. Advertisements designed to get you to try some sort of "natural" such-and-such for some particular ailment are all over the Internet and social media. The problem is that many of these products are untested, unregulated, may not contain what they claim to contain, could be dangerous, and may simply end up being a rip-off. It is important to learn more about complementary therapies in order to choose those that have some track record of safety and efficacy.

When starting a complementary therapy, a stroke survivor may find it a little awkward or even uncomfortable. This reaction is normal, but the more he takes part in a particular therapy, the more comfortable he will become with it. Over time, he can determine for himself whether he experiences any benefit from engaging in this treatment method.

TAI CHI

The Chinese martial art of tai chi has a long history of use in self-defense training, but in recent years, the health benefits associated with tai chi have been the primary driver of interest in its practice. Tai chi involves coordinated movements that are often described as circular, continuous, controlled, gentle, slow, smooth, and soft. Many forms of tai chi can be done in a chair, or holding on to a chair, and movements that are too difficult can be modified.

There is a growing amount of research on the positive impacts of tai chi on health. (Many of these studies are summarized in *The Harvard Medical School Guide to Tai Chi* by Peter Wayne, PhD, with Mark L. Feurst.) Tai chi has been found to improve balance, reduce falls, decrease pain, curb cardiovascular disease risk, boost psychological well-being, and improve sleep problems. Unfortunately, it has not been studied extensively in association with stroke treatment. A recent review of studies testing the effects of tai chi after stroke found only two small randomized controlled trials of stroke patients. In the larger study, only 145 participants were enrolled and each person was assigned to tai chi or group exercise classes or usual care for twelve weeks. In terms of depression, physical quality of life, and psychological quality of life, the research showed no difference between groups.

If a stroke patient wishes to give tai chi a try, he will need to find a class, teacher, and form of tai chi that fit his needs. In addition, he should discuss with his therapist whether or not it he is ready to do tai chi. It is important to be aware that there is no certification process for tai chi teachers in the United States, so anyone can call herself a teacher. A potential student should talk to potential instructors in advance of committing to a class, or have his loved one do this research on his behalf. Do these teachers focus on the self-defense aspect of tai chi or are they more interested in helping people with health issues? With whom have these teachers studied tai chi? For how long have they studied tai chi? As there are many different forms of tai chi, a stroke patient or his loved one may want to visit a class to see if the form being taught and the teaching style are a good match for his needs. A good place to start looking for a teacher is a local Department of Parks and Recreation or community center. (For more information, see page 289 of the Resources.)

YOGA

Originating in India, yoga has been practiced for thousands of years and is now known internationally for its physical, mental, emotional, and spiritual benefits. Of course, if you are at all familiar with yoga, you may be wondering how a stroke survivor with physical limitations could possibly contort his body into some of the poses taught in yoga. The fact is that yoga can be adapted for almost any individual.

A review of randomized controlled trials of yoga after stroke found three small studies of fair quality. The studies did not show any differences in the qualities of life, depression levels, or anxiety levels of its subjects, although one study showed improvement in memory. Nevertheless, when participants were asked how they felt, those who had done yoga reported feelings of increased strength, flexibility, balance, and walking ability. They also said they felt calmer, more confident and energetic, less stressed, and in a better mood. Lastly, they said their minds felt more connected to their bodies.

Yoga may help rewire the brain after a stroke because it requires the practitioner to pay close attention and concentrate. Yoga's slow, deliberate motions may encourage the brain to heal. A patient's walking may improve as he is able to take longer and better coordinated steps. If he has significant weakness and cannot participate in gentle yoga exercises, he could still concentrate on the meditative and mental aspects of the practice. His breathing may improve as he practices breathing slowly and deeply during his yoga sessions. He may also be able to do some stretching exercises.

A stroke patient or one of his loved ones should ask his healthcare provider if yoga is safe for him, and if she could recommend a yoga instructor who has special training and experience in helping stroke patients. A local Department of Parks and Recreation may also offer information on yoga classes for stroke patients. (For more information, see page 289 of the Resources.)

MUSIC THERAPY

Music therapy may also help a stroke survivor in his recovery. No, a music therapist is probably not going to teach a patient how to sing or play an instrument—that's music education. Music therapy is the use of music to treat patients who have motor, speech, cognitive, or mood problems. It is another complementary way to attempt to diminish the effects of a stroke.

Music therapy with rhythmic auditory stimulation, which uses the rhythm of music, has been shown to improve recovery of walking and arm movements after stroke. In addition, training with musical instruments can improve the speed, precision, and smoothness of arm movements after stroke. Melodic intonation therapy, which uses the melody and rhythm of music to train speech production, has been shown to improve the ability to speak in individuals with aphasia. Finally, different forms of active music therapy, such as singing or music composition, have been shown to improve mood and increase social interaction among individuals with stroke.

Although better studies on music therapy are required, present research on this subject indicates that music therapy may improve walking, speed of repetitive arm movements, communication, and quality of life. Therapy that uses music with a strong beat may be more effective than interventions that use a strong beat without music, while treatment delivered by a trained music therapist may be more effective than treatment delivered by other professionals.

A stroke survivor or his loved one may ask members of his medical team if they could recommend a good music therapist. A music therapist will choose specific music tailored to the needs of a client, so she should be informed of the type of music he loves. Does he love marches? Songs with words? Hymns? Dance music? She should know the songs that once energized her patient, the ones that got him moving.

Movement is strongly affected by music. If a patient is struggling to walk, his favorite music may help him walk more normally, as long as it has a good beat. One good option would be *The Battle Hymn of the Republic,* which has a steady rhythm. Perhaps a patient could walk and sing to his high school or college fight song. If he is unable to walk, he could try to stand and sway to music. If he is able, he could even try a few dance steps. If he is in a wheelchair, he could sway, clap his hands, tap his foot, tap his fingers, or just listen.

As mentioned in Chapter 7, some stroke survivors who cannot use normal speech actually find they can sing instead. A patient's ability to speak common phrases in a sing-song manner may provide him with a means of communication.

Music therapy also stirs the senses and emotions. As a result, it can be a powerful tool in recovery, lifting mood and easing anxiety. This is an important aspect of music therapy, as stroke patients often face anxiety and depression after experiencing a stroke. When a stroke survivor feels better emotionally, he is more likely to engage in thera-peutic exercises such as occupational, physical, or speech therapy. He is also more likely to feel energetic enough to prepare healthy meals and have an appetite to enjoy these nutritious foods.

ACUPUNCTURE AND ACUPRESSURE

Chinese medicine teaches that there are channels of energy running in patterns through the body and skin, and that these channels can be activated through *acupuncture,* which refers to the placing of very fine stainless steel needles at specific points on the body (called *acupuncture points,* or *acupoints*) to help the body heal. Acupuncture has been used in China for thousands of years to promote health and well-being, prevent illness, and treat various medical problems, including stroke.

Acupressure uses fingertips rather than needles to stimulate acu-points on the skin. The same targets as acupuncture are stimulated with pressure using fingers or thumbs. Sometimes acupressure is used alongside aromatherapy. (See page 122.) It is also used alongside traditional therapy such as physical or occupational therapy.

The World Health Organization recognizes the use of acupuncture for digestive, respiratory, neurological, and muscular disorders. But what about stroke? Acupuncture therapy has been used to treat stroke survivors in China, Korea, and Japan for centuries. Scientists in these countries have studied the use of acupuncture to treat stroke patients, finding that stroke patients who received acupuncture therapy also tended to get better sooner, perform better in self-care, require less nursing and rehabilitation therapy, and use less healthcare dollars than those who did not receive this therapy. In one Korean study of stroke patients with weakness, acupressure was reported to improve upper arm movement, increase participation in daily living activities, and decrease depression.

A review of thirty-one trials of acupuncture for rehabilitation after stroke found that subjects who received acupuncture also experienced benefits in activities of daily living (such as bathing, dressing, and feeding) and specific neurological aspects, including strength, cognition, depression, swallowing, and pain. The quality of these trials, however, was considered low, so additional rigorously designed randomized controlled trials are needed.

IS CHIROPRACTIC CARE SAFE FOR STROKE SURVIVORS?

Chiropractic care refers to the manipulation of the musculoskeletal system, especially the spine, to heal the body. More than 27 million Americans have chiropractic adjustments each year for various medical problems. Chiropractors must be licensed in their state. Obviously, many people are pleased with their care, but does chiropractic care work for stroke survivors, and is it safe?

Chiropractic manipulations may help patients with low back pain, and some chiropractors work with traditional doctors to relieve pain in other parts of the body. Nevertheless, there are no studies to support the use of chiropractic manipulations in stroke treatment. In fact, manipulation of the neck has been associated with stroke in several studies, particularly the high-velocity neck manipulation commonly practiced in chiropractic care, which can cause a vertebral artery dissection. As described earlier in this book (see page 33), a dissection (a tear in a blood vessel) can cause a stroke, especially in young adults and middle-aged adults. In fact, dissections account for 8 to 25 percent of strokes in people younger than forty-five years of age. When a tear forms in an artery, clots form at the site of the tear, causing the artery to narrow and therefore increasing the risk of stroke. For this reason, the American Stroke Association released a scientific statement to inform people of the statistical association between neck manipulation and stroke.

A review of fifty-nine randomized controlled trials examined the use of acupuncture in treating lifestyle risk factors after stroke. While acupuncture had seemingly no effect on blood pressure after stroke, subjects who received ear acupressure for smoking dependence also reported smoking fewer cigarettes each day than those who received sham acupressure, in which pressure is used but not on the proper acupoints. Compared to sham acupuncture, those who received acupuncture for obesity had lower waist circumference than those who received the sham treatment. Unfortunately, the methodological quality of these studies was found to be poor, so additional randomized controlled trials are needed.

In recent years, Western medicine has begun using acupuncture as a complementary treatment. Western doctors have concluded that acupuncture needles may stimulate the nervous system to release chemicals in the muscle and brain.

Acupuncture or acupressure in stroke therapy may not be covered by Medicare but may be covered by some private health plans. A member of a stroke patient's healthcare team may be able to recommend an acupuncture or acupressure therapist. It is important to find a practitioner who is well trained and experienced.

MASSAGE

Massage refers to the rubbing and kneading of muscles and joints. It has not been studied in stroke patients in randomized controlled trials, but it has been studied for other conditions such as depression, anxiety, and blood pressure.

A rehabilitation facility sometimes has a massage therapist as part of its treatment team. If not, a team member may be able to provide a recommendation. Before a stroke patient takes advantage of massage therapy, he or his loved one should ask his doctor if doing so would be appropriate at that time. She may want him to wait, as blood clots may exist that he doesn't want to disturb with massage. She may advise against a massage therapist massaging the neck area because she would not want clots in neck arteries to be released and cause another stroke. If a patient is on blood thinners, she may want him to avoid deep massage because of the possibility of bruising.

Medicare does not cover massage therapy, but some additional health insurance policies may cover some of the cost. All in all, massage may offer benefits to stroke survivors just as it does to folks who are well. And it feels wonderful.

AROMATHERAPY

Aromatherapy refers to the use and application of essential oils extracted from plants to improve mood and for certain medicinal purposes. These oils give a plant its "essence"—its unique scent and flavor—and include peppermint oil, lemon oil, lavender, and many others. While these oils have been used since ancient times, they have been studied more in the last century. Aromatherapy has been used for relaxation, easing anxiety, relieving depression, enhancing alertness, improving sleep, or relieving pain.

After the essential oil of a plant has been extracted from its flowers (e.g., lavender), leaves (e.g., eucalyptus, geranium), or stems (e.g., lemongrass), it is added to a "carrier oil" (e.g., grapeseed oil, olive oil, coconut oil, or almond oil), diluting it and making it ready for use. An essential oil may be applied to the skin, through which it is absorbed into the bloodstream, or vaporized and then inhaled, a process by which it is absorbed by the small blood vessels in the nasal passages. Oils may be applied through massage, vaporizers, baths, creams, or lotions.

Each essential oil is thought to have a certain effect on the user. Essential oils such as chamomile, sandalwood, and lavender are said to relieve stress, improve mood, and enhance relaxation. Jasmine and lemon oils may improve depression and mood. Patients often say they "just feel better after aromatherapy." Aromatherapy's overall rewards may be increased when the positive chemical effects of an essential oil are coupled with the benefits of massage, if this is the chosen form of application. Touch is powerful and healing in itself.

Some companies sell essential oils to be taken orally, but in many cases these have not been studied for their safety and effectiveness. One form of oral lavender oil, however, which comes in capsules of 80 to 160 mg, has been tested in clinical trials and was found to relieve anxiety in patients diagnosed with an anxiety disorder. Essential oils have not been studied in stroke survivors; therefore, their effects in individuals with stroke are unknown.

Anyone interested in trying aromatherapy in any form should talk to his healthcare provided about it first. He should ask his doctor or pharmacist whether a particular essential oil could affect any of the prescription drugs he has to take. For example, peppermint oil can increase the concentration of some medications in the blood, including the antidepressant amitriptyline and the statin simvastatin.

Like most "natural" therapies, aromatherapy can cause side effects from mild to severe. Yes, you can overdose and get too much of a good thing. The most common side effect is skin irritation with swelling, redness, and sometimes tiny blisters. But other side effects are possible, such as allergic reactions (sometimes severe), seizures, lung and breathing problems, vomiting, or even kidney damage. A person trying an essential oil for the first time should test it by rubbing a drop or two into a small area of his skin or taking in one breath or two of the vaporized oil. If no negative reaction occurs, he could try using more the next day.

HYPERBARIC OXYGEN THERAPY

Hyperbaric oxygen therapy, or HBOT, refers to exposing a patient to 100 percent oxygen in a whole-body chamber under extra atmospheric pressure. You may have heard about deep sea divers who get decompression sickness—the "bends"—and are treated successfully using HBOT. It is also used to help heal persistent wounds. Essentially, once a person is placed in an HBOT chamber, the amount of pure oxygen in the chamber is increased three or four times per square inch, so as he breathes, he will receive a higher and higher level of concentrated oxygen until the chamber reaches 100 percent.

The Food and Drug Administration has approved the use of HBOT in the treatment of several medical conditions, including carbon monoxide poisoning, decompression sickness, burns, and gangrene. The FDA has not approved HBOT for use in stroke patients, however, because there simply isn't any data currently available to support it. Scientists have postulated that high levels of oxygen might act as a neuroprotectant in the early stages of stroke, protecting brain cells from dying and possibly facilitating recovery after stroke, but thus far only a few very small studies have been conducted to test this hypothesis, and these did not show any positive results. Additional studies are needed to determine if HBOT may truly be a worthwhile aid in stroke recovery.

CONCLUSION

Complementary therapies may be helpful in stroke recovery. Since they have not been studied in large, rigorous clinical trials, they should not be used instead of prescribed therapies. Complementary therapies should always be discussed with and approved by a patient's healthcare provider before use. It is important for her to have a full understanding of his medical status so she can advise and treat him properly during his recovery.

PART III

Stroke Prevention

9

*M*anaging
Risk Factors

As explained in Chapter 2, there are risk factors for stroke that you cannot change, such as your age and race, but there are many risk factors that you can reduce or eliminate entirely to prevent a TIA or stroke. In fact, modifiable factors such as high blood pressure, abdominal obesity, smoking, physical inactivity, and poor diet account for the overwhelming majority of strokes around the world. Other common risk factors that may be adjusted include type 2 diabetes and abnormal cholesterol.

Additional issues that contribute to stroke risk include irregular heart rhythm, hormonal therapy or contraceptive use, depression, heavy alcohol use, illicit drug use, recent heart attack, migraines, pregnancy, and sleep apnea. This chapter discusses methods to improve or even eliminate many risk factors for stroke. These methods include taking certain medications and making particular lifestyle changes, including increasing physical activity, following a healthy diet, and stopping smoking.

MEDICATION

There are a number of medications that can do wonders to lower or even reverse many of the risks for stroke. Of course, pills will not solve every problem, and it is important for stroke survivors to understand what a medication is designed to do, when a medication is best taken, and the potential side effects of a medication. If a patient has more than one healthcare provider, he should be sure that each provider knows exactly which medications and supplements he is taking in order to avoid any harmful interactions.

Atrial Fibrillation

In individuals with atrial fibrillation (afib, or AF), the two upper chambers of the heart, known as the *atria*, receive signals to beat irregularly. When this happens, the atria do not squeeze properly, but instead quiver. As a result, blood is more likely to remain stagnant, or pool, in the atria, leading to the formation of clots. The left atrium has a little outpouching called the left atrial appendage. Most clots form in this structure. If a clot dislodges, it can be thrown into the arteries leading to the brain, causing an ischemic stroke. Untreated atrial fibrillation increases the risk of stroke by a factor of approximately five. Blood-thinning drugs such as warfarin, apixaban, dabigatran, rivaroxaban, and edoxaban can reduce the risk of ischemic stroke due to atrial fibrillation by making it less likely for a clot to form in the heart.

Atrial fibrillation often does not cause any symptoms. When it does, patients often report that they feel their hearts pounding or "flip-flopping" in their chests. They also may complain of fatigue, generalized weakness, decreased exercise endurance, dizziness, and shortness of breath.

Some people go in and out of irregular rhythm in what is called *paroxysmal atrial fibrillation*. It is important to know that both intermittent (paroxysmal) and persistent atrial fibrillation increase stroke risk; therefore, a patient should be on a blood thinner regardless of which type he has. Blood thinners are also recommended for individuals with a related condition known as *atrial flutter*, which is characterized by the atria squeezing in a rhythm that is a bit less chaotic than they would in connection with atrial fibrillation. Despite this difference, patients with atrial flutter are also at a high risk of stroke.

There is a procedure called *left atrial ablation* that is meant to treat the symptoms of atrial fibrillation, such shortness of breath or feeling the heart pounding in the chest), although it does not reduce the risk of stroke, so a patient would still require blood thinners to prevent a stroke even after having had this procedure.

There are several options when it comes to blood-thinning medications. The one that has been studied and used for many years is warfarin (commonly known under the brand name Coumadin). Patients who are on warfarin have to get their blood levels checked regularly, as the medication has to be adjusted to ensure proper dosage. Foods such as leafy green vegetables can affect blood levels of warfarin, so patients on this medication should either limit consumption of these foods or simply make sure they eat the same amount of leafy greens every day.

In recent years, numerous *direct oral anticoagulants* (DOACs) have been approved for use in stroke prevention in connection with certain atrial fibrillation patients. These DOACs include apixaban, dabigatran, rivaroxaban, and edoxaban. Their advantages include not requiring patients to have their blood levels monitored, not being affected by diet, and possibly offering a lower risk of bleeding (particularly bleeding in the brain) than warfarin.

For stroke survivors who cannot be on long-term blood thinners but who can use them for a short time, another option is available. It is an implanted device called the Watchman, which blocks off the left atrial appendage. Implanting this device does not involve open heart surgery. It is simply guided into the heart through a flexible tube (i.e., catheter) that has been inserted into a vein in the groin region. The implant is introduced through the right atrium and passed into the left atrium through a small puncture hole. Once the position is confirmed, the device is released and the catheter is removed. A patient with this implant will need to take both warfarin and aspirin for several weeks to reduce the risk of clot formation on the device.

Cholesterol

Statin drugs, particularly atorvastatin, have been associated with lowering the risk of stroke. If a person has had a stroke, his healthcare provider will likely prescribe a statin medication. If a stroke patient has high triglycerides, his healthcare provider may prescribe another medication such as niacin or fenofibric acid. It is important to note that other types of medications may have interactions with statins. Thankfully, certain non-drug methods, such as diet and exercise, can also improve cholesterol levels.

Clot Formation

In a patient with an ischemic stroke, one of the most important medications to prevent another stroke is a medication to reduce clot formation, called an antithrombotic. Antithrombotics include antiplatelet medications (such as aspirin, clopidogrel, dipyridamole, and cilostazol) and anticoagulants (such as warfarin, apixaban, dabigatran, rivaroxaban, and edoxaban). Anticoagulants are often called "blood thinners." For particular conditions such as an irregular heart rhythm (atrial fibrillation) or a clot in the heart, an anticoagulant will be recommended to lower the risk of another ischemic stroke. For most strokes, though, an antiplatelet will be recommended. All antithrombotics can increase the risk of bleeding and result in prolonged or excessive bleeding. The increased bleeding risk can be mild, causing easy bruising or frequent or prolonged nosebleeds; or severe, such as a gastrointestinal bleed (which can cause blood in the stool, black stools, or vomiting blood) or a bleed in the brain (hemorrhagic stroke). Despite these increased risks associated with antithrombotics, the benefits of these medications in regard to stroke reduction outweigh their possible negative side effects.

A patient on antithrombotic medication should keep in mind that certain prescription medications, over the counter medications, and supplements can increase bleeding risk. These include non-steroidal anti-inflammatory medications (e.g., ibuprofen, naproxen, and diclofenac), antidepressant medications (e.g., fluoxetine, sertraline, citalopram, and escitalopram), medications used to suppress the immune system (e.g., methotrexate, azathioprine, and mycophenolate), and supplements (e.g., fish oil, St. John's wort, ginkgo biloba, and garlic). A patient should always check with your pharmacist or medical provider before starting new medications or supplements.

Depression

Depression is both a risk factor for stroke and a common effect of stroke. As mentioned in Chapter 2, symptoms of depression may include feelings of sadness, sleep disturbances such as insomnia or oversleeping, poor concentration, feelings of guilt, appetite issues (either not having an appetite or craving and overeating unhealthy foods), low energy levels, lack of interest in doing formerly enjoyable things, slow speech or functioning, and thoughts of suicide. In addition, depressed individuals do not recover from stroke as well as those who are not depressed. It is therefore important to recognize and treat depression promptly in people at risk of having a stroke and people who have already had a stroke.

A healthcare provider will be able to offer many different types of medications and counseling to treat depression. If one medication doesn't help, a different one may be prescribed. The most common medications for treating depression are called *selective serotonin reuptake inhibitors* (SSRIs). Examples include fluoxetine (Prozac), sertraline (Zoloft), citalopram (Celexa), escitalopram (Lexapro), paroxetine (Paxil, Pexeva), and vilazodone (Viibryd). Serotonin is a chemical messenger in the brain that sends signals between brain cells. It has many functions, including regulating feelings of well-being and happiness, appetite, digestion, sleep, memory, and sexual desire and function. Individuals with depression tend to have low levels of serotonin in the brain. SSRIs block the reuptake of serotonin by cells, resulting in higher levels of serotonin in the brain. For this reason, SSRIs have been extremely successful in treating the symptoms of depression.

It is important to note that SSRIs can take a few weeks to work and often need to be increased in small increments until they successfully treat symptoms. Many people are resistant to taking antidepressants because they think doing so will turn them into completely different people or make them feel like zombies. These outcomes are inaccurate. Antidepressants can make individuals with depression feel more like themselves. SSRIs can have side effects, however, such as dry mouth, headache, restlessness, weight loss or gain, excessive yawning, dizziness, or tremor, but often these side effects go away after a few weeks.

Antidepressants may improve weakness after stroke. A small study in France of stroke survivors with moderate to severe weakness gave half the participants the SSRI antidepressant fluoxetine and the other half a placebo (inactive pill). At three months, the group who had received the antidepressant showed more improvement in strength than the group who had received the inactive pill. A much larger trial in the UK gave half its subjects fluoxetine and the other half an inactive pill for six months. At six months there was no difference in disability between groups, but fluoxetine had helped prevent depression. More patients who had received fluoxetine, however, developed bone fractures. For this reason, antidepressants are not typically prescribed unless there is a diagnosis of depression.

Type 2 Diabetes

Controlling blood sugar and A1c levels is an important part of preventing a first stroke or avoiding recurrent strokes in the future. There are numerous medications for controlling blood sugar, and a healthcare provider's prescription will be based on the specifics of a particular case of high blood sugar.

A medication known as pioglitazone has been studied in stroke survivors with insulin resistance, which occurs before the onset of type 2 diabetes. In a trial involving stroke or TIA patients who did not yet have diabetes but had insulin resistance, the risk of stroke or heart attack was lower among patients who received pioglitazone than among those who received a placebo. Pioglitazone was also associated with a lower risk of type 2 diabetes but with higher risks of weight gain, edema, and fracture. Due to the elevated risk of fracture associated with this medication, it is not often used. There are also, of course, non-pharmaceutical methods that may be used to lower blood sugar, including exercise, diet, and sleep. All these methods should be employed to lower stroke risk.

It's important to check for diabetes or prediabetes in order to spot it early and start treating it as soon as possible. Once type 2 diabetes is diagnosed, one must carefully control blood sugar levels. Doing so can reduce the risk of stroke and heart attack. In people with type 2 diabetes, it is also critical to control blood pressure and cholesterol to reduce stroke risk. Research has shown that bringing blood glucose levels down to a moderate target reduces the risk of future strokes. On the other hand, while reducing sugars to an even lower target helps eye and kidney health, it is not likely to reduce the risk of stroke further.

SPECIAL CONCERNS FOR DIABETICS

Patients with type 2 diabetes are at increased risk of having a stroke. Due to their high blood sugar levels, type 2 diabetics have a special constellation of biological factors that can increase their chances of experiencing a stroke. Effective strategies to reduce stroke risk in diabetics include:

- Preventing or delaying the onset of type 2 diabetes through diet, exercise, and medication.

- Preventing hardening of arteries by controlling high blood pressure, high blood cholesterol, and high blood sugar, as well as by not smoking.

- If an ischemic stroke has occurred, using a blood-thinning medication to discourage blood clots from forming.

- If a patient's neck artery has signs of plaque on an ultrasound, CT scan, or MRI, he or his loved one should ask his healthcare provider about "cleaning out" or stenting the artery to reduce his risk of having a stroke.

High Blood Pressure

As mentioned earlier, high blood pressure is the biggest risk factor for stroke, and controlling blood pressure should be the most important goals for most stroke survivors. After a stroke, particularly a stroke due to atherosclerosis, or plaque in the arteries, a patient will most likely be placed on blood pressure medication. Types of blood pressure medications that have been shown to reduce the risk of a second stroke include thiazide diuretics (such as hydrochlorothiazide), angiotensin converting enzyme (ACE) inhibitors (such as lisinopril or benazepril), and calcium channel blockers (such as amlodipine, verapamil, or nifedipine).

In addition to blood pressure medication, there are non-pharmaceutical ways to lower blood pressure, including exercise, behavioral therapy, diet, weight loss, and lifestyle changes, which are discussed later in this chapter.

Thiazide Diuretics

Thiazide diuretics, also known as *water pills,* are blood pressure medications that directly affect the kidneys, lowering their ability to reabsorb sodium and chloride (the compound of which is known as salt), which the kidneys release into the urine. Sodium and chloride then take water from the body to increase urine flow. This effect on the kidneys leads to an increase in urination and a reduction in fluid accumulation and swelling, also known as *edema.* As the amount of fluid flowing through the blood vessels decreases, so does the pressure on blood vessel walls, thus lowering blood pressure.

ACE Inhibitors

ACE inhibitors work by preventing the formation of a hormone called *angiotensin II.* Angiotensin II is involved in numerous activities that increase blood pressure, such as holding on to sodium and chloride (and thus retaining water), and constricting, or squeezing, arteries. By blocking angiotensin II, ACE inhibitors lower blood pressure.

Calcium Channel Blockers

Calcium channel blockers prevent calcium from entering the cells of the heart and blood vessel walls, thus relaxing the arteries. Blood pressure then drops because blood flows more easily through these relaxed arteries.

Combination

The combination of a thiazide diuretic and ACE inhibitor, in particular, reduces the risk of another stroke dramatically. While other medications can lower the blood pressure, they have not been found to reduce the risk of another stroke in a patient who has had a TIA or stroke. If a patient is on a different type of blood pressure medication (for example, a beta-blocker, such as atenolol or metoprolol), he or his loved one may want to ask his healthcare provider if he can switch to a pharmaceutical regimen that has been studied in relation to stroke, specifically a regimen made up of a combination of a thiazide and ACE inhibitor or a calcium channel blocker.

Being an Advocate

A healthcare provider's choice of blood pressure medication for a stroke patient will likely depend on other medical conditions this patient may have. It is important to remember that not all clinicians are aware of the best medications for stroke prevention, so strokes patients should not be afraid to act as their own advocates or have their loved ones act as their advocates. If a patient happens to experience any side effects from a medication, his healthcare provider needs to be made aware of this fact. A patient should not, however, stop taking a medication without discussing doing so with his healthcare provider.

Monitoring Blood Pressure at Home

High blood pressure levels can occur with no outward signs. One way to maintain control of blood pressure is to measure it regularly, become aware of normal fluctuations throughout the course of the day, keep track of blood pressure levels, and discuss these levels with a healthcare provider. Blood pressure monitors can be bought at local pharmacies without a prescription. There are typically two types: one that is placed on the wrist, and one that is placed on the upper arm. The upper-arm version tends to have more accurate readings. If a stroke survivor cannot take his own blood pressure, a loved one could do it for him. Regularly checking, recording, and discussing blood pressure with his healthcare provider are incredibly important methods to prevent another stroke.

Smoking

For many people, breaking the smoking habit is extremely difficult. In spite of all the deadly diseases associated with smoking, which include stroke, some stroke survivors can't stop lighting up. Quitting smoking may be a difficult goal to achieve, but there is help. Medications such as varenicline, nortriptyline, and buproprion can be effective tools in stopping smoking, as they are designed to relieve withdrawal symptoms. A healthcare provider will be able to recommend a pharmaceutical aid.

Another option is *nicotine replacement therapy*, or NRT. Nicotine is the addictive chemical in tobacco that causes smokers to crave another cigarette after a period of not smoking. Nicotine replacement therapy provides alternative ways to deliver low doses of nicotine, keeping cravings under control and allowing a smoker to refrain from smoking. When it comes to NRT, there are a variety of choices. There are nicotine patches, gums, inhalers, nasal sprays, and lozenges. NRTs are available without a healthcare provider's prescription, but anyone considering using a particular NRT should check with his health insurance to see if it is covered. Some plans will pay the cost of an NRT if it has been prescribed by a doctor.

In addition to these smoking cessation aids, behavioral therapy can be a helpful tool in trying to kick the habit. (See page 141.)

Weight

Obesity is the most prevalent chronic disease in the United States, with 41 percent of women and 38 percent of men being obese. As discussed in Chapter 2, obesity increases the risks of high blood pressure, abnormal cholesterol, type 2 diabetes, heart attack, stroke, and a variety of other conditions. There have been hundreds of well-designed studies on interventions to lose weight. The majority of these are behavioral interventions such as a reduced calorie diet and increased physical activity. Medications for weight loss can be considered for those people who don't lose 5 percent of their weight with an intensive behavioral program. Whenever medications are used, however, they should complement, not substitute, a healthy diet and regular physical activity.

There are several medications approved by the FDA for weight loss. They work in different ways, including suppressing appetite (making a person less hungry), enhancing satiety (making a person feel full), reducing blood sugar levels (thus reducing the production and storage of fat), and blocking fat absorption. The most common method used is suppression of appetite. One such appetite-suppressant medication is phentermine-topiramate (Qysmia). Phentermine-topiramate is a combination pill of a sympathomimetic medication (with properties similar to amphetamines) and a medication used for epilepsy and migraine. Although its safety in the setting of stroke is not known, it is probably best to avoid this medication after a stroke or TIA, as it revs up the sympathetic (fight or flight) system. In addition, medications with amphetamine properties can be associated with *reversible vaso-constriction syndrome*, resulting in sudden narrowing of the arteries of the brain, causing strokes.

Naltrexone-bupropion (Contrave) is a combination medication used for weight loss. Both naltrexone and bupropion act as appetite suppressants. Buproprion alone is also used for treating depression. Both bupropion and naltrexone have been shown to help with weight loss, but when used together, they have a bigger effect. One of the most serious possible side effects of this medication is an increased risk of depression and suicide. Liraglutide (Victoza), a medication that is injected daily under the skin, is used for both type 2 diabetes and weight loss. It reduces blood sugar spikes in the blood by increasing insulin release when a person eats. It also delays movement of food in the stomach (gastric emptying), thus creating a feeling of fullness. Liraglutide has some serious potential side effects, however, including pancreatitis (inflammation of the pancreas) and thyroid cancer. For this reason, its use should be discontinued if less than 5 percent of body weight is lost after twelve weeks of therapy.

Finally, orlistat works by blocking some of the fat that is eaten from being absorbed by the body. Xenical is the prescription-strength form of orlistat. Alli is the brand of orlistat available without a prescription.

PHYSICAL ACTIVITY

Modern medicine has come up with a variety of medications to reduce a person's stroke risk, but people should not depend on drugs alone. There are many non-drug approaches to decrease stroke risk, and there's no reason why non-medical methods shouldn't be used in combination with medical treatments, as long as a healthcare provider is consulted first. These approaches include lifestyle changes, including dietary modification, physical activity, quitting smoking, and reducing alcohol use.

Physical activity or exercise programs undertaken after TIA or stroke have been found to improve stroke risk factors by lowering blood pressure, blood sugar, and bad cholesterol (LDL) levels, and increasing good cholesterol (HDL) levels. Exercise promotes weight loss and increases strength and endurance. It also reduces levels of stress, anxiety, and depression, and improves sleep. Clearly, exercise is a powerful tool to lower several risk factors for a TIA or stroke.

When it comes to exercise, there are several types to consider: aerobic, muscular strength and endurance, flexibility, and neuromuscular. *Aerobic exercise* increases your heart rate and makes you breathe in more oxygen, thereby benefiting your heart, brain, and muscles. Fast walking, biking, dancing, and tennis are aerobic activities. Aerobic activities have numerous benefits for stroke survivors. They increase walking speed and efficiency, improve exercise tolerance, promote independence in activities of daily living, strengthen muscles, improve cognition (the ability to think and process information), and improve heart health.

Muscle strength and endurance activities include resistance training of the upper and lower extremities and trunk using free weights, weight-bearing or partial weight-bearing activities, elastic bands, spring coils, pulleys, or circuit training. Muscle strength and endurance activities promote independence in activities of daily living and job functions, and make it easier to lift or carry objects.

Flexibility exercises include stretching. Stretching helps with range of motion in affected limbs, reduces the risk of injury, and promotes independence in activities of daily living, and prevents the development of contractures, which are defined by the shortening and hardening of muscles.

Neuromuscular activities include balance and coordination activities such as tai chi, yoga, the use of paddles and sport balls, and interactive computer games. These activities enhance balance, quality of life, and mobility. They also decrease fear of falling and improve safety while doing activities of daily living.

Setting Up an Exercise Program

A stroke patient's healthcare provider should decide the best time for him to resume physical activity, and exercise should be customized for him, taking into account his exercise tolerance, stage of recovery, environment, available social support, physical activity preferences, specific impairments, and activity limitations. The goal should be to engage in aerobic exercise three to five times a week for twenty to sixty minutes per session, strength training two to three days a week (one to three sets of ten to fifteen repetitions of eight to ten exercises involving the major muscle groups, as tolerance permits), stretching two to three times a week, and neuromuscular activities two to three times a week. If you have had a stroke, you may react to this advice by saying, "I can hardly stand up! I'll never be able to do that!" Remember, however, that this advice is simply a goal. A healthcare provider or physical therapist will be able to tailor an exercise program to your abilities.

Stroke survivors need to start slowly and then gradually increase the time of the sessions and the intensity of exercise. For example, if he is able to stand and walk, his short-term goal may be to stand and walk for two minutes. His long-term goal may be to walk briskly for thirty minutes three to four times a week. If he is in a wheelchair, just pushing the chair as far as he can on his own will increase his heart rate and breathing and strengthen his arms.

In addition to performing aerobic exercise, patients who engage in regular strength, flexibility, and coordination-building physical activities may recover motor skills more quickly while reducing their chances of falling. A physical therapist can recommend balance and strength exercises.

Exercising doesn't have to mean running a marathon or biking ten miles. A patient should set reasonable goals so that he stays motivated and encouraged by his progress.

Blood Pressure

High blood pressure may be much better controlled when blood pressure medication is combined with aerobic exercise. In some cases, with exercise, a lower dosage of medication can be used. It is important to note that a person should never lower the dosage of or stop taking a blood pressure medication without speaking to a healthcare provider first, of course.

Blood Sugar

Besides lowering blood pressure, exercise can also lower blood sugar. When a person exercises, his muscles "burn" glucose, or sugar, for energy, reducing the sugar levels in his blood. Exercising can also lead to weight loss, which also lowers blood sugar. With exercise and a healthy diet, a person with prediabetes may avoid progressing to full-blown diabetes.

Depression

Exercise can improve symptoms of mild to moderate depression and is sometimes as effective a treatment as antidepressants. Exercise is often recommended along with prescription medications to relieve depression. Perhaps it's the endorphins that are released during exercise that affect brain chemistry, lifting depression. The chemical structure of endorphins and effects are similar to the drug morphine, making them able to relieve pain naturally and make you feel better. It is often difficult for a person who is depressed to get himself "in gear," so to speak, but if he is able to do it, exercise will make him feel better.

Sleep

The sleep benefits of exercise are just another reason to get moving. Aerobic exercise not only shortens the time it takes to fall asleep but also enhances sleep quality. It is even all right to exercise close to bedtime. As long as the exercise isn't too intense, exercising before going to bed is fine. Insomniacs, however, should not exercise before bed.

Weight

Exercise promotes the burning of calories, which is a necessary part of weight loss. The more intense the exercise, the greater number of pounds will be lost. The act of walking slowly burns calories, but walking quickly burns even more. Biking on level ground will encourage weight loss, but biking on hills will lead to greater weight loss, as it burns more calories. If a stroke patient, or anyone, would like to lose weight, he should set a realistic goal with the input of his healthcare provider and choose an enjoyable exercise plan to reach it.

Stress

Stress is the normal response to various fear-inducing events in the environment. Your body responds to stress by generating a "flight or fight response" that enables you to deal with a crisis by either fighting it or running away from it, producing the hormones norepinephrine and cortisol in the process. These hormones enable you to deal with an emergency. Unfortunately, your body reacts in the same way to a truly life-threatening event, such as being chased by a large animal (as our ancestors were), as it does to an overwhelming nuisance, such as being stuck in heavy traffic and realizing you may be late for an important meeting as a result. The latter type of stress is extremely common, which is why so many people are under chronic stress.

And what happens to a person who is under chronic stress? The previously mentioned hormones increase blood pressure, raise blood sugar levels, and are likely to make a person overeat, causing obesity. As recently mentioned, exercise causes the body to release endorphins. Endorphins help with stress relief. A mildly stressed person would benefit from walking, riding a bike, or going to the gym with a friend. A person with chronic stress may benefit from engaging in vigorous activity three to four times a week if possible.

PHYSICAL TRAINERS

If a person is struggling with exercise, obesity, high blood sugar, depression, or quitting smoking, a physical trainer might be just what he needs. Physical trainers can be physical therapists, occupational therapists, gym trainers, or former athletes. A good physical trainer can motivate you to exercise and help you identify exercises you like and can do. She will offer a regular exercise schedule, which will promote a healthy lifestyle. A physical trainer may be needed only for a few sessions, after which working out with a friend or alone would be fine.

Starting an Exercise Program

Exercise makes you feel better in every way, with the exception of a few sore muscles. Exercise can help alleviate all kinds of physical and mental issues, so a stroke patient or at-risk individual should start an exercise regimen as soon as possible. Stroke survivors will need to build up to a reasonable exercise routine. They should talk to their doctors and physical therapists about the types of exercises they should do and the lengths of time for which they should do them. Once a stroke patient makes exercise part of his daily routine, he will come to enjoy it and discover how it can provide him with so many positive health benefits.

BEHAVIORAL THERAPY

Behavioral therapy refers to methods that help you change bad habits and replace them with healthy ones. We all exhibit different behaviors and habits, which we acquire as we grow up and move through life. While some patterns of behavior may be influenced by our genes, most are based on our childhoods and family experiences—what our parents told us and demonstrated by their behaviors; behaviors we experienced as teenagers under strong peer pressure; and behaviors we witnessed as adults at work and during our leisure time with friends and family.

If your parents were in the habit of overeating and often chose unhealthy sugary, salty, and fatty foods, you likely became addicted to sugary, salty, and fatty foods at an early age. As a teenager, you may have hung out with peers who smoked and perhaps did drugs, so to look "cool" you smoked and took drugs, too, and quickly became addicted to these harmful substances. If your close adult friends drink to excess, you may go along with the crowd but over time discover you are unable to stop, resulting in an alcohol addiction.

The older we get, the more "set in our ways" we become. The fact is that we find great comfort in our habits. We all know we should eat a healthier diet, stop smoking, drink less, get more sleep, and exercise more, but we avoid making healthy choices because we see them as too difficult, putting them off for another day. In addition, many of us are unconsciously addicted to our many unhealthy behaviors. Just thinking about any changes makes us anxious. Then, suddenly, wham, a stroke occurs, and we learn that our choices likely contributed to its occurrence—and now is the time we must change our life-long bad habits. While it is not an easy task, it not an impossible one either. Through various methods of behavioral therapy, millions of people have changed their habits.

The right behavioral therapy can help you deal with your smoking addiction, tendency to eat unhealthy foods, or habit of drinking too much alcohol. It can also help you handle stress better. Behavioral therapy can be conducted by different types of professionals—a healthcare provider, nutritionist, physical trainer, psychological therapist, social worker, trained group leader, or even a pet, provided that pet is a great listener!

There are many behavioral therapies, but there is no one behavioral therapy that works for everyone. The Resources section at the back of this book provides many sources of information on behavioral therapy and ways to break your addictions. (See page 290.)

■ ONE-ON-ONE BEHAVIORAL THERAPY

One-on-one therapy occurs between a patient and a therapist only. The benefit of one-on-one therapy is that a therapist can focus on her patient and her patient's issues completely and without distraction. One-on-one therapy also offers a patient more privacy. One-on-one therapy may be more expensive, but health insurance may cover it.

Alcoholism

Behavioral therapy for alcohol abuse is usually conducted by psychiatrists, psychologists, or trained alcoholism counselors. Many people who drink to excess deny they have problems. Social alcoholics, while able to "handle their liquor," see drinking as a means to relax. The fact is that excessive consumption of alcohol may lead to a stroke. If a stroke has occurred, it is important for the stroke survivor to recognize the connection between drinking and stroke and do something about it. There are a wide variety of one-on-one therapies available to help an individual quit drinking, including cognitive behavioral therapy (CBT) and motivational interviewing.

Cognitive behavioral therapy (CBT) is a problem-focused and action-oriented form of therapy. It helps subjects develop skills to alter the way they react to situations. *Motivational interviewing* is a technique that gets a subject to examine how he feels about any changes he is hoping to make. By asking pointed questions, a therapist can elicit a patient's uncertainties and hesitancies, which may stop him from making these changes. Motivational interviewing can help a patient make changes to habits that may not serve him well. It may take time to find the approach that works for a particular individual.

Depression

Cognitive behavioral therapy has also shown to be effective in treating depression. A cognitive behavioral therapist will often ask a patient to discuss a stressful or distressing situation. She will then help the patient identify cognitive distortions that may have framed how he reacted to the situation, and help him to frame the situation differently. A *cognitive distortion* is a belief, thought, or attitude that causes a person to perceive reality inaccurately. This negative outlook on reality can have a profound impact on mood. Examples of cognitive distortions include always having to be "right," blaming others, discounting positive events, emotional reasoning (e.g., "I feel stupid, therefore I must be stupid"), labeling (i.e., attributing a person's actions to his character), magnifying or minimizing events, overgeneralizing, personalizing, "black or white" thinking (e.g., thinking a person is either good or bad), and making "must" or "should" statements (e.g., "I should have recovered from my stroke by now").

Supportive therapy may also be used to reduce or relieve symptoms of depression and distress. In this form of therapy, a therapist simply reinforces a patient's healthy and adaptive patterns of thought. *Person-centered therapy* may also be employed to alleviate depression. This refers to therapy in which a therapist relates to her client without hiding behind a professional façade; offers acceptance to a patient without expressing disapproval, judgment, or advice; and expresses empathy. This method encourages a patient to feel comfortable enough to express himself without fear of judgment. A therapist does not offer solutions to the patient, but rather helps him arrive at solutions for himself. Finally, in addition to its use in the treatment of alcoholism, motivational interviewing can also be used to address depression.

Stress and Anxiety

One-on-one behavioral therapy may help reduce stress and anxiety. Relief from stress and anxiety may come from seeing a psychiatrist, psychologist, social worker, minister, or even a massage therapist. It could even come from the comfort of having dog or cat. Of course, pets can't give advice, but they are great listeners, have endless time, and are warm and loving.

A psychiatrist may want to prescribe medication to treat stress and anxiety, while a psychologist would help her patient identify why and where he feels stressed or anxious. She may recommend exercise, tai chi, or yoga. (See page 289.) Some psychologists may even suggest meditation CDs or apps, which a patient can use to reduce anxiety and stress and even improve sleep.

APPS

There are many apps out there to help people do all kinds of things. Some apps provide a live online counselor to lead a one-on-one session. Other apps may have a fixed but effective program. There are apps to help you stop smoking, lose weight, relax, or even set you up with a healthy diet—the list is endless! The Resources section at the end of this offers a few examples of such apps.

Weight

If an individual needs to lose weight, he may meet one-on-one with a doctor, dietitian, or nutritionist. This professional should have a degree in nutrition science or be a registered dietitian. This weight loss professional will weigh her client at each visit, at which reasonable, realistic, achievable goals may be discussed with her. Beyond that, many professionals have their own approaches to working with their clients. A client should make sure he feels comfortable working with his professional of choice.

One last point: While there are many ways to lose weight and counting calories is important, never forget that the quality of the foods consumed is just as important as the calorie count. (See Chapter 10 on page 153.)

Finding a Behavioral Therapist

As you may have noticed, numerous professionals can provide behavioral interventions, including physicians, psychologists, nutritionists, occupational therapists, physical therapists, exercise physiologists, nurses, and community health workers. One-on-one therapy can help a stroke survivor or at-risk person reduce many of his stroke risk factors by helping him lose weight, stop drinking excessively, stop smoking, set up an exercise regimen that he would enjoy, choose a healthy diet, or lower his stress, anxiety, or depression. A good therapist will help her patient determine what triggers him to eat too much, drink too much, or smoke and replace these activities with healthier alternatives.

Anyone searching for the right behavioral therapist should start by inquiring with a healthcare provider and then speaking to family or friends to see if any of them have had good experiences. There are many behavioral therapists out there. If one doesn't work out, it is important to realize that there are others available. Finding the right person is important.

■ GROUP THERAPY

Some effective behavioral therapies take place in a group environment. Group settings include gyms, health facilities, colleges, high schools, recreation centers, and places of worship. The advantages of group therapy are that it costs less and attendees get to learn together, make friends, and share their experiences—both their failures and successes. Group therapy provides peer support, allows for problem-solving with others who are facing similar challenges, and encourages sticking to goals. Group therapy is one place where peer pressure is a good thing. A person is more likely to make changes in his life when other people are trying to do the same thing.

Alcoholism

For someone who has been drinking excessively and cannot stop doing so, group behavioral therapy is available. No doubt, the most well-known group therapy for alcoholism is the twelve-step program Alcoholics Anonymous, or AA. Research has shown the benefits of twelve-step programs. Alcoholics are sure to find a lot of support for stopping drinking and staying sober at AA meetings.

Exercise

Group exercise is a good way to make friends and ensure that you follow your exercise regimen. If you are a stroke survivor, finding an exercise group for stroke survivors would be ideal, as it would be sensitive to the needs of people who may have physical limitations. A group leader such as a physical trainer or physical therapist would determine exercises that are appropriate for the whole group.

Water aerobics at the local YWCA might work well for you if you are a stroke survivor. The water helps with balance and gives some resistance as you walk to exercise your muscles. It helps you stretch your muscles and improve your coordination. And it can be fun in a group setting. Gyms today often include a pool. A water aerobics instructor may be a swimming teacher or a physical therapist. After the class ends, a stroke survivor may want to buy a membership so he can swim a couple of times a week, gradually building up his endurance. Choosing a variety of group exercises may keep him interested—for example, swimming twice a week, working out at the gym twice a week, and walking or biking on the other days.

Some hospitals and rehabilitation centers also have Wellness Centers, which can include a gym, cooking classes, peer support groups, or other key resources for patients.

Food Preparation

A stroke patient or his loved one should look for cooking groups that meet to prepare healthy meals and snacks that he can eat after he makes them. The leader of a cooking group may be a nutritionist or a local cook interested in healthy foods. Cooking groups discuss ingredients—how to choose them at the grocery store and store them at home, and how to prepare them. Attendees will learn healthy cooking ideas from their teacher and from each other. There is a good chance they will also make friends with similar interests in eating healthy food and have a good time. Cooking classes may be offered by a local hospital, healthcare facility, school, or parks and recreation department. Of course, stroke patients should steer clear of classes that use ingredients such as sugar, corn syrup, excessive salt, or "bad" fats.

Smoking

Group behavioral therapy can also help you stop smoking. The American Lung Association has been helping people quit smoking for over thirty–five years through its "Freedom from Smoking" efforts. The association runs stop smoking clinics throughout the United States. Each group consists of eight to sixteen smokers plus a trained person to lead eight sessions. Group therapy is great because members can encourage each other. They can discuss problems they are having with others who are having similar problems. These sessions may also provide motivating information to help a smoker decide to quit. The group will discuss what triggers cigarette cravings, strategies for avoiding these triggers, and how an individual can change his response to these triggers.

Changing Bad Habits

Group behavioral therapy can be the key to abandoning bad habits and choosing healthy alternatives. Taking part in certain group activities can even be fun. There are many groups out there that offer people an opportunity to make friends with others who are interested in adopting a healthier lifestyle.

MEDITATION

Meditation is a method to achieve a state of calm awareness. It has been practiced for thousands of years and has been woven into a number of religions, cultures, relaxation techniques, and types of therapy. There are many forms of meditation, including mindfulness meditation, focused meditation, and transcendental meditation. The benefits of meditation are both physical and mental. The practice of meditation has been shown to reduce cardiovascular risk factors. A healthcare provider can offer advice on this subject. She may even be able to suggest meditation teachers. There are even apps for meditation. (See page 291 of the Resources section.)

Blood Pressure

While other relaxation techniques have largely been unsuccessful in reducing blood pressure in studies, meditation has had some promising results. In one study, unmedicated patients with high blood pressure either engaged in meditation or did not. Those who meditated lowered their blood pressures by about 10 percent. Meditation is especially helpful because it requires no equipment, can be done anywhere, and is generally inexpensive to learn. It also does not produce the side effects that may come with pharmaceuticals. (We do not, however, recommend meditation as a substitute for necessary medication.)

Blood Sugar

Meditation may also help lower blood sugar levels. In one study, patients with prior heart attack were divided into two groups—one group meditated for six months while the other group did not. At the end of the study, patients who had meditated had reductions in their blood sugar and hemoglobin A1c readings.

Depression, Anxiety, and Pain

In a review of numerous trials that included more than 3,500 participants, researchers reported small to moderate improvements in anxiety, depression, and pain in those who meditated. Meditation may even reduce or eliminate the need for anti-depressant medication.

GOOD FOODS VS BAD FOODS

Most of us eat what we like, and usually the foods we prefer are those we have grown used to eating. As children, for good or bad, we eat what our parents give us. As we get older, we become more discriminating, consuming foods that we think taste good, satisfy our hunger, and in many cases, are convenient to cook or to pick up at a local restaurant or market. Of course, if the majority of these foods were good for us, perhaps we could have fewer health issues—from strokes and heart attacks to type 2 diabetes and cancer. But, as we know, our poor diet underlies our world's health crisis.

The truth is that many of the foods we like—sweet cereals and crunchy, salty snacks, for instance—were designed by manufacturers to turn on our taste buds but offer little to no real nutritional value. In addition, many of these foods are highly addictive, from the fizzy highly sweetened sodas we drink to the luscious desserts we ask for after eating a full meal. And, of course, all that clever advertising convinces us that certain foods will make us happy. Just think of all the TV commercials that show a young couple in love sharing sweet, colorful foods, giving the unspoken message that if you eat these foods, then you, too, will feel loved. Or people at a party who look happy eating their favorite snack foods with all their friends participating, conveying the message that these snack foods will make you socially comfortable and popular. All these ads are little more than scams to help you stay addicted to bad foods.

When we are young, our diet usually seems to create no problems, but as time marches on, our bodies begin to suffer the consequences of poor eating. Stroke is one of these consequences, and statistics, unfortunately, don't lie. Strokes are occurring more often in younger people, indicating that their diets are so unhealthy that they run the risk of having a stroke or other illnesses much sooner than the children of a generation prior.

By understanding which foods are good and which foods are bad, you can gain control of what you consume. You will have to answer the question, "Shall I decide to change my diet and choose a longer, healthier life or shall I continue as I've been doing all my life but face illness, disability, and an earlier death?" It is a question only you can truthfully answer.

This book can help those who wish to give up lifelong food addictions and habits. As you will read in the next chapter, a lack of the right nutrients may be at the root of modern illness, along with eating bad foods, which are discussed in Chapter 11 (see page 175). Chapter 12 (see page 196) discusses good foods that provide all the essential nutrients. Finally, Chapter 13 (see page 215) identifies healthy foods that can be used to create meals and snacks.

SUPPLEMENTS

Supplements include vitamins, minerals, essential fatty acids, herbs, and other natural nutrients that are taken by capsule, pill, powder, liquid, or as an herbal tea—they supplement the diet. You may be thinking, "If I were to eat a healthy diet, why would I need supplements?" There is an answer to this question.

First, the suggested amounts of nutrients, known as the Recommended Dietary Allowance (RDA), were formulated by the United States Department of Agriculture to meet the needs of 97 to 98 percent of healthy Americans; they may be inadequate for you. Second, nutrient absorption declines with age. So, the nutrients you consume at age twenty are absorbed to a greater degree than the nutrients you take in at age sixty. Third, the pesticides and herbicides used to grow our foods, plus environmental pollution, increase our needs for vitamins and minerals, which detoxify these harmful chemicals.

Fourth, as you begin to exercise you may need more vitamins and minerals. Fifth, if you eat a poor diet, then you may need supplements. (But don't think you can eat as you please and make up for poor food choices by taking supplements. A healthy diet is very important.) Sixth, taking certain supplements may improve your blood sugar or blood pressure. (But don't expect a certain supplement to keep you from having a stroke—there are so many factors that play a role in why you may be at risk of a stroke.) Finally, our foods are grown in fields that are often depleted of essential nutrients from over-farming.

In turn, our foods are often nutritionally deficient. If you can find locally grown organic foods, they may be a better option.

The next chapter provides more information about supplements—which ones decrease stroke risk factors according to scientific studies, why they work, and how much to take. It also explains which supplements have not been helpful in preventing strokes or in aiding in stroke recovery.

LIFESTYLE TIPS

While this entire chapter is essentially about achieving a healthy lifestyle, it is important to take a moment and outline how to lead a healthy lifestyle every day, which can be done by observing the following guidelines:

- Eat nothing but healthy foods, as described earlier in this chapter and in the chapters that follow.

- Exercise each day, even if it means going for only a short walk.

- Enjoy the outdoors and the sunshine, and appreciate talking to neighbors.

- Maintain a normal weight—a BMI of 18.5 to 24.9 kg/m^2 (see pages 28 and 29)—by eating only good foods and exercising.

- Manage stress through meditation, yoga, tai chi, or exercise.

- Don't smoke, take drugs, or drink too much alcohol.

- Spend less time in front of the TV, using a computer, or playing on a smart phone or tablet.

It's also important to keep mentally stimulated, whether it is by reading interesting books or meeting with friends to have interesting discussions. Some people may wish to participate in their places of worship and learn more about their faiths.

Even though Americans have the highest incomes of wealthy nations, they have shorter life expectancies than the inhabitants of many other high-income nations. According to Harvard health researchers, the impact of practicing a healthy lifestyle as previously described could add as much as fourteen years to the life expectancy of women at age fifty, and about twelve years to the life expectancy of men at age fifty. Not only does a healthy lifestyle lead to a longer life, but quality of life is also improved.

CONCLUSION

Managing risk factors for stroke, which include high blood pressure, high blood sugar, type 2 diabetes, abnormal cholesterol, obesity, a sedentary lifestyle, poor diet, and depression, is possible. While medication can be effective in controlling some risk factors, non-drug approaches including exercise, diet, meditation, and behavioral therapy can also help lower stroke risk. The Resources section on page 286 can help you find more information on a specific approach.

Even with the right resources, it's not always easy to take the first step. But this step must be taken. It leads to the realization that a new and better life is closer than it once seemed to be.

10

$\mathcal{N}$utrients That Protect

Many nutrients are known to protect against stroke and heart disease. They protect cells against oxidative stress, improve blood vessel health, help control cholesterol, and perform other important functions that can aid stroke prevention. The more a patient and his caregivers know about these important nutrients, the better choices they will make when selecting foods to eat or supplements to take.

This chapter discusses vitamins, minerals, essential fatty acids, and other nutrients that stroke patients need to protect their brains and blood vessels. The role each of these nutrients plays in protecting against future strokes is explained.

A healthy eating plan that includes a wide range of wholesome foods is vital for good health. Although Americans have access to the largest supply and variety of foods in the world, too many of us make poor food choices, and consequently, our diets are low in a number of critical substances.

The following nutrients help protect all your cells, but especially those of the cardiovascular system and brain. Armed with this knowledge, a patient or his loved one will be able to work confidently with a healthcare provider to make important decisions about diet and supplements.

VITAMINS

A nutrient is a substance that is required to function and sustain life. Vitamins are organic nutrients (meaning they contain carbon atoms) that an organism must acquire to survive because it cannot create them biologically in sufficient amounts or at all. Vitamins are considered micronutrients because they are needed in only small quantities. Vitamins contribute to good health by regulating metabolism, which refers to the chemical reactions that occur to maintain the life of an organism. These reactions include all the chemical changes that nutrients undergo from the time they are absorbed until they either become a part of the body or are excreted from the body. Thirteen vitamins are generally recognized as being essential, meaning that they are needed for the body to function: vitamins A, C, D, E, K, and all the B vitamins.

Vitamins are grouped into two categories, water-soluble and fat-soluble. As their name implies, water-soluble vitamins dissolve in water. They must be taken into the body daily because they are excreted in the urine on a regular basis—sometimes in as little as two hours—instead of being stored for future use in fatty tissue. Included in this vitamin group are the B vitamins and vitamin C.

Advice for Caregivers
CHOOSING FOODS CAREFULLY

As soon after your loved one's stroke as possible, while he is still in the hospital or rehab, encourage him to start choosing foods that will help him heal. As soon as he is able to chew and swallow, he should consume whole oats, brown or wild rice, whole grain barley, whole wheat bulgur, and whole rye as cereal, bread, or pasta. His diet should also include lots of fruits and vegetables, unprocessed nuts, skim milk and unsweetened low-fat yogurt, and lean meat, poultry, and fish. (See Chapter 12 on page 196 for details on recommended foods.)

If he is having swallowing and chewing problems, ask his health-care providers if these options would be suitable: oatmeal, farina (Cream of Wheat), unsweetened applesauce, canned unsweetened soft peaches, cooked carrots, cooked sweet potato, unsweetened yogurt with soft fruit, poached eggs, meatloaf, cooked chicken, and fish. Encourage him to choose protein at every meal. Suggest he skip the sweet desserts, soft drinks, and candy, and encourage visitors to bring him healthy foods.

Fat-soluble vitamins dissolve in fat rather than water and are stored in the body's fatty tissue and liver. They include vitamins A, D, E, and K. The human body and brain need both water-soluble and fat-soluble vitamins to perform normally. This chapter outlines the most important vitamins in stroke prevention.

Vitamin A and the Carotenoids

Vitamin A, a fat-soluble vitamin, plays a role in many biological functions. For example, it helps maintain healthy skin, eyes, teeth, bones, soft tissue, and mucous membranes. As a powerful antioxidant, it is involved in reducing inflammation and fighting free-radical damage.

The average diet provides two types of vitamin A. A group called retinoids comes from animal sources. This type of vitamin A is pre-formed—in other words, it is ready for use by the body. Because vitamin A is fat-soluble and not readily excreted from the body, it can accumulate and create an imbalance, which could become toxic when doses are extremely large.

The second class of vitamin A provided by the average diet is known as the carotenoids. These nutrients come from plants. There are over sixty carotenoids found in food, the most famous of which is beta-carotene. Of all the carotenoids, only a few of them—beta-carotene included—are converted by the body into active vitamin A and then act like pre-formed vitamin A. (The other carotenoids also have important functions in the body.)

So, should a stroke patient supplement his diet with vitamin A or beta-carotene? It is fine if vitamin A is included as one of the ingredients in a general multivitamin pill, but there seems to be no evidence that supplementing stroke patients with vitamin A prevents another stroke. An increased dietary intake of beta-carotene and related nutrients, however, does seem to reduce the risk of stroke and other cardiovascular diseases. It is usually best to get beta-carotene and its related nutrients from nutrient-packed food sources, such as carrots, sweet potatoes, sweet red peppers, winter squash, dark green leafy vegetables, cantaloupe, and apricots.

In terms of beta-carotene supplements, it is important to note that an increased risk of lung cancer in smokers has been linked to taking beta-carotene supplements but not to consuming beta-carotene in the diet. In addition, a supplement of beta-carotene will not include the other important carotenoids found in foods, which can help protect against stroke. In this case, a stroke patient should let food be his medicine.

B Vitamins

The nutrients known as the B-complex vitamins are grouped together based on their common sources, their close relationship in vegetable and animal tissue, and their functional relationship. These water-soluble substances include vitamins B_1 (thiamine), B_2 (riboflavin), B_3 (niacin), B_5 (pantothenic acid), B_6 (pyridoxine), B_{12} (cobalamin), biotin, choline, folate, inositol, and para-aminobenzoic acid (PABA). B vitamins are found naturally in meat, dairy, leafy greens, peas, and whole grains.

While a certain B vitamin may be taken individually to treat a deficiency, as is often the case with vitamin B_{12}, B vitamins are so interrelated in function that it is often recommended they be taken together in a combination supplement.

Unfortunately, modern Western diets often don't provide enough B vitamins, as they are high in processed foods rather than vitamin B-rich whole grains and greens. In addition, certain medications (such as antacids, metformin, and seizure medications) can block absorption of B vitamins in the digestive tract.

Studies show that consuming a diet rich in fruits, vegetables, and whole grains reduces the risk of having a stroke. A person who follows the AHA diet (see Chapter 12 on page 196) will get a rich supply of B vitamins, and because these nutrients are water-soluble, there is no chance of overdosing on them.

Does taking supplements of B vitamins reduce a person's risk of stroke? Research studies suggest it may in certain people, particularly those who live in countries that do not fortify grains with B vitamins. A combination of folate (folic acid), vitamin B_6, and vitamin B_{12} lowers an amino acid called *homocysteine*, which is occasionally elevated in stroke patients. Homocysteine can increase stroke risk by making the blood more prone to clotting and accelerating plaque buildup (atherosclerosis) in arteries.

There have been several clinical trials that studied B-vitamin supplementation in stroke prevention, the results of which were mixed. While a few of the trials showed reductions in stroke risk, others did not, and there were adverse events reported in some trials, such as a higher risk of cancer in the group that had received the vitamin therapy. Further research is needed to determine which patients may benefit from supplementation. Given the inconsistent evidence from the trials, doctors do not routinely screen for homocysteine levels in the blood and generally do not prescribe B_6, B_{12}, or folate to stroke patients. In addition, in the United States, it is rare for people to have high homocysteine levels, as B vitamins are added to grains. To get all the B vitamins needed to combat modern diseases, an individual should carefully follow the AHA diet.

ANTIOXIDANTS AND FREE RADICALS

Antioxidant nutrients play an important role in preventing strokes, but what exactly are antioxidants and why are they so valuable?

When the body's cells use oxygen to generate energy, free radicals, also known as oxidants (molecules with an uneven number of electrons) are generated. Free radicals can steal an electron from other molecules, causing those molecules to become unstable. Think of a free radical as a highly reactive molecule that acts like a "spark," causing other molecules to become "sparks," which lead to other "sparks" in a chain reaction. Free radicals can be beneficial or harmful. At low levels, they play a role in sending messages between cells and help the immune system. At high levels, however, they can result in a condition known as oxidative stress, in which cells sustain substantial damage.

These unstable molecules can also form when toxic chemicals such as those in tobacco smoke or other air pollution enter the body. Free radicals can rupture cell membranes, causing the loss of cellular components and making the cell useless. They can even cause changes in DNA. The chemicals in a ruptured cell leak into surrounding tissues, damaging them. This process is associated with numerous disorders, including high blood pressure, type 2 diabetes, stroke, heart disease, arthritis, cancer, Parkinson's disease, and Alzheimer's disease.

We depend on special enzymes (proteins) manufactured by the body and natural chemicals in our foods called antioxidants to neutralize free radicals. Antioxidants neutralize free radicals by giving these unstable molecules an electron without becoming unstable themselves. Think of antioxidants as fire extinguishers that put out the "sparks." Vitamins such as C and E; carotenoids such as beta-carotene; minerals such as zinc and selenium; and other nutrients help defend the body from free radical damage.

It's important to understand that antioxidants can be easily used up or depleted. This is why it is crucial to eat a nutrient-rich diet that provides an abundance of antioxidants. Finally, you may be wondering: If antioxidants play such a crucial role in good health, are supplements recommended? Antioxidant supplements are obtained by extracting them from natural foods or chemically synthesizing them. They do not have the same composition as antioxidants found in foods and have not been shown to lower stroke risk in any trial. In addition, if taken in large quantities, antioxidant supplements actually pose a danger of accelerating oxidative stress—the opposite of their advertised effect. Since supplements are not regulated in the same way medications are, and as quality can differ from one batch to the next, it is best to rely on diet to ensure good antioxidant levels in the body.

Vitamin C

Vitamin C, or ascorbic acid, is a water-soluble vitamin and antioxidant that performs a number of important functions in the body. This nutrient builds and maintains collagen, a protein necessary for the formation of the walls of the tiny blood vessels known as capillaries. A reduction in collagen levels can therefore lead to these blood vessels being weakened. Fortunately, vitamin C is found in high amounts in a number of fruits and vegetables, including oranges, kiwi, papayas, berries, tomatoes, bell peppers, broccoli, dark leafy greens, and green peas.

Studies have shown that people who consume a diet rich in vitamin C and those who have high levels of vitamin C in the blood also have a lower risk of stroke than people who consume less vitamin C and have low levels in the blood. Of course, high levels of vitamin C in the blood are associated with a greater intake of fruits and vegetables, so the risk reduction may be due to a combination of nutrients, not just vitamin C. A high dose of vitamin C supplementation (500 mg a day) has been shown to decrease blood pressure mildly, but little is known about the long-term risk of vitamin C supplementation, so it is not generally recommended for blood pressure control. In addition, taking vitamin C supplements does not seem to lower stroke risk.

Because vitamin C is water soluble, it's important to eat vitamin C-rich foods several times a day. Studies have confirmed that vitamin C is flushed from the body in less than three hours, so it should be consumed often.

Vitamin D

You are probably aware of the important role vitamin D plays in building strong bones and teeth, but do you know that low levels of vitamin D have been associated with high blood pressure, heart disease, stroke, and cancer? Low levels of vitamin D can alter several pathways associated with plaque formation, leading to heart disease and stroke. In addition, vitamin D has antioxidant and possible anti-inflammatory properties that appear to make it important in the prevention and slowing of cardiovascular disease.

Several studies have shown that individuals with low blood levels of vitamin D have higher stroke rates than individuals who have high levels of vitamin D. Low levels of vitamin D are also related to poorer physical recoveries and more cognitive impairment after a stroke. Furthermore, as you know, the risk of depression is high in patients who have had a stroke, and this may be related to their lower vitamin D values. Vitamin D levels in stroke patients who had experienced depression prior to having a stroke have been shown to be lower than those of stroke patients who had not experienced depression.

Few foods provide vitamin D. It is found in mushrooms, egg yolks, liver, and oily fish. It is also found in vitamin D-fortified milk, yogurt, margarine, and orange juice. The human body produces its own vitamin D when sunshine strikes the skin, but with the current emphasis on less sun exposure because of skin cancer concerns, many

Americans tend to avoid the sun, a habit that greatly decreases the body's production of vitamin D.

Considering these factors, perhaps it should not come as a surprise that, even though vitamin D is a fat-soluble nutrient and can be stored in the body, more than 42 percent of US adults (82 percent of African Americans) are deficient in vitamin D. If you have low levels of vitamin D and are able to be outside, then try to spend fifteen to twenty minutes (less if you have very fair skin) a day in the sun, but be sure to use sunscreen. Everyone should try to avoid sunburn, which can cause skin cancer.

So far, no study has shown that vitamin D supplementation lowers stroke risk or improves outcomes after stroke. It may be reasonable to measure vitamin D levels and start supplementation with D_3 if levels are low. If a stroke patient's vitamin D levels are found to be low and he will be spending most of his time indoors, it is likely that his doctor will also recommend he take supplements of vitamin D_3. A daily dose of 2,000 IU to 3,000 IU may be beneficial, but every person is different. His vitamin D levels should be checked again after two or three months to see if they have increased substantially or if his dose needs to be adjusted.

Vitamin E

Vitamin E, a fat-soluble vitamin, is a strong antioxidant that protects cells, tissues, and organs from oxidative stress. In particular, vitamin E decreases free radicals formed by oxidation of essential fatty acids (EFAs). (Learn more about EFAs on page 165.) Vitamin E also helps provide protection against the damaging effects of many environmental toxins in the air, food, and water, including those in tobacco smoke.

Despite the antioxidant effects of this nutrient, vitamin E supplements do not seem to improve stroke or other cardiovascular events, and may even increase the risk of hemorrhagic stroke in some patients with high blood pressure. In light of this information, it seems wise to get vitamin E from the diet. Foods high in vitamin E include almonds, spinach, sweet potatoes, avocados, wheat germ, butternut squash, and olive oil.

Advice for Caregivers
MEASURING BLOOD LEVELS OF NUTRIENTS

A caregiver of a stroke patient should consider asking his healthcare provider to measure a few of the nutrients mentioned in this chapter if she has not already done so, as they are frequently low in stroke patients. If levels are low, supplementation may be warranted.

MINERALS

A mineral is a naturally occurring substance that is solid and inorganic, meaning it does not contain carbon. The body needs certain minerals in order to function, which may be attained from food or supplements.

Minerals may be divided into two groups: macrominerals and microminerals. Macrominerals are needed by the body in large amounts. They include calcium, chloride, magnesium, phosphorus, potassium, sodium, and sulfur. Microminerals, on the other hand, are needed by the body in small amounts, which is why they are also referred to as trace minerals. They include chromium, cobalt, copper, fluoride, iodine, iron, manganese, molybdenum, selenium, and zinc. It should be noted that the amount needed in the body is not an indication of a mineral's importance. The following minerals are involved in cardiovascular health.

Calcium

You are no doubt aware that calcium is important in building and maintaining strong teeth and bones. You may not know that your muscles, heart, and nerves also require calcium to function normally. Calcium plays a role in the multiple pathways that lead to an ischemic stroke. Too much calcium, however, is also harmful.

A person who consumes two servings of dairy products—cheese, milk, or yogurt—each day should get enough calcium. Dark green leafy vegetables such as broccoli and kale, and fish with edible soft bones are also sources, as are fortified foods and beverages—those foods to which manufacturers have added vitamins and minerals—such as cereal, fruit juice, soy milk, and other milk substitutes. (Be sure to read the labels.)

If a stroke patient doesn't (or can't) eat foods or drink beverages that are good sources of calcium, calcium supplements (usually given with vitamin D) may be recommended. Calcium carbonate is the cheapest form, but the pills are often gigantic. Calcium citrate is better absorbed and can be purchased as a powder, which can be mixed into water or juice. A patient's doctor will determine the daily dosage to be taken.

Chromium

Chromium is a trace mineral. Needed only in small amounts, it stimulates the activity of enzymes that are essential in carbohydrate, lipid, and protein metabolism. It is involved in the breakdown of glucose (sugar), and also appears to enhance the effectiveness of insulin, thereby increasing the transport of glucose into the cells. Since type 2 diabetes, a condition characterized by poor glucose metabolism, is a risk factor for stroke, adequate levels of chromium could play an important role in stroke prevention.

According to a review of numerous studies on this topic, however, chromium supplements seem to have limited effectiveness in controlling blood sugar, so supplements are not routinely recommended for diabetics to improve glucose metabolism. In addition, no studies have found that chromium supplements help prevent stroke or alter recovery after stroke.

As is the case with many other nutrients, acquiring this mineral from whole food sources may be the best way to enjoy its benefits. Chromium is found in a variety of foods, including vegetables, fruits, meats, and seafood, but most of these sources contain only small amounts of the nutrient. The foods highest in chromium include shellfish, pears, Brazil nuts, and tomatoes.

Copper

Although required in only minute amounts, this mineral performs a variety of important functions. It aids in energy production, assists in thyroid function, decreases inflammation, serves as a component of enzymes, and more.

Research, however, has shown high levels of copper in the blood of stroke patients. Therefore, a stroke survivor should not take copper supplements. The foods highest in copper are liver and oysters, but this mineral is also found in nuts and seeds, legumes, cherries, avocados, eggs, whole grains, and poultry. Most common foods contain only a small amount of copper, so getting copper in the diet shouldn't pose a problem.

If a patient has macular degeneration, he may be taking a nutritional supplement known as AREDS to treat it. This supplement contains copper to balance its high zinc content, but it is still fine for stroke patients to take.

Magnesium

Magnesium is needed by the body and affects a wide variety of biological functions. Among its many roles, magnesium has been shown to lower blood pressure, improve blood flow, and improve metabolic syndrome. Moreover, magnesium helps the body maintain proper blood sugar levels; therefore, it may be associated with prevention of type 2 diabetes. Because high blood pressure, metabolic syndrome, and elevated blood sugar are risk factors for stroke, it makes sense that obtaining sufficient magnesium is important for cardiovascular health.

It should be no surprise that higher magnesium dietary intake is associated with lower stroke risk. A stroke survivor's doctor should measure his magnesium level. If it is low, his healthcare provider may decide to give him magnesium supplements.

Many Americans do not get enough magnesium in their diets. Only 25 percent of US adults get the recommended amount of magnesium. Foods high in magnesium include dark leafy greens, almonds, pumpkin seeds, whole grains, beans, fish, avocados, bananas, and yogurt. Moreover, because the body requires and uses magnesium for so many functions, it's easy to deplete stores of this nutrient. For this reason, it may be prudent to take a daily magnesium supplement, the dosage of which will be dependent on need and should be discussed with a healthcare provider. The use of magnesium supplements may be prohibited, however, if a stroke patient has kidney disease, which can prevent the body from eliminating excess amounts of magnesium. Lastly, if supplementation leads to diarrhea or abdominal pain, usage should be discontinued.

Potassium

Like magnesium, potassium is involved in many important functions of the body, including fluid balance, nerve signaling, heartbeat, muscle contractions, and blood pressure. As you know, reducing blood pressure is one of the keys to reducing stroke risk.

Unless a doctor prescribes potassium supplements, it is best to get this nutrient from the diet. In general, a diet that provides an abundance of fruits and vegetables will help ensure a healthy amount of this mineral. The foods highest in potassium include avocados, acorn squash, spinach, sweet potatoes, dried apricots, pomegranates, white beans, and bananas.

Of course, it is possible to get too much of a good thing. The body's potassium-sodium balance is delicate, and too much potassium can cause serious side effects, including a fatal heart rhythm. If a stroke patient has kidney disease, which can prevent his body from eliminating excess amounts of this mineral, his potassium needs should be discussed with his doctor.

Selenium

Selenium is a trace mineral that is essential in minute amounts to make the body perform optimally but is toxic if too much is consumed. Selenium as part of other molecules has important antioxidant effects. Selenium levels in soil vary considerably around the world and within the United States, but most Americans get all the selenium they need from the diet. By eating a variety of fruits, vegetables, whole grains, dairy products, seafood, lean meats, poultry, eggs, and nuts, an individual can acquire sufficient selenium. Just one warning: Brazil nuts are much higher in selenium than other foods, so they should not be eaten every day—occasionally is fine, though, and beneficial.

Selenium supplements do not seem to reduce the risk of cardiovascular disease and may increase the risk of type 2 diabetes, elevated total cholesterol, low HDL, and high triglycerides. Although selenium may be studied in the future as a substance that protects brain cells, also known as a *neuroprotectant,* supplementation is not recommended after stroke.

Zinc

Although this micromineral is needed in only small amounts, zinc plays a multitude of roles in the body. It is a constituent of at least twenty-five enzymes involved in digestion and metabolism. Zinc is an antioxidant and also has anti-inflammatory effects. The list of zinc's functions goes on and on.

What is zinc's role in ischemic strokes? While it is not completely clear, in one Chinese study of individuals with high blood pressure, those with higher zinc levels had lower rates of hemorrhagic stroke.

A wide variety of foods contain zinc. Oysters, red meat, and poultry are the richest sources, but other good sources include beans, nuts, whole grains, dairy products, and fortified breakfast cereals.

ESSENTIAL FATTY ACIDS

The fats known as essential fatty acids (EFAs) are necessary for optimal health. Moreover, these fats, when chosen carefully, can be protective against stroke and cardiovascular disease.

Essential fatty acids are termed "essential" because they are required for good health but cannot be made by the body and therefore must be acquired from certain foods or supplements. Omega-3 fatty acids, the most famous of which are long-chain n-3 polyunsaturated fatty acids (n-3 PUFAs) eicosapentaenoic acid (EPA), docosapentaenoic acid (DPA), and docosahexaenoic acid (DHA), are the building blocks of cell membranes. Along with omega-6 fatty acids, they keep the watery material around cells separate from the watery contents of cells, and they are also responsible for the structural integrity of each cell's components. Omega-3s also have anti-inflammatory and antioxidant effects. They reduce the risk of blood clots by preventing platelets from sticking together, and they reduce blood pressure by encouraging blood vessel walls to relax.

In three large studies that followed different groups of people over many years (the Nurses' Health Study, Cardiovascular Health Study, and Health Professionals Follow-Up Study), higher levels of DPA and DHA in the blood were associated with lower risk of ischemic stroke. Levels of EPA, however, did not have an effect on stroke risk. It is important to note that both EPA and DHA lower very high triglyceride levels and increase good cholesterol (HDL) levels, which are beneficial effects, but they also increase bad cholesterol (LDL) levels.

Combination EPA-DHA supplements typically come in the form of fish oil capsules. A daily fish oil supplement of 1,000 mg to 2,000 mg may be beneficial, but a patient should discuss any omega-3 supplements with his healthcare provider before starting a daily regimen.

The body needs both omega-3s and omega-6s to function properly. A review of nineteen studies of omega-6 fatty acids showed that they may reduce risk of heart attacks and lower total cholesterol. According to the review, however, they did not demonstrate any effect on stroke risk, triglycerides, good cholesterol (HDL), or bad cholesterol (LDL). Omega-6 fatty acids are found in sufficient amounts in vegetable oils such as corn, soy, safflower, and sunflower. Most Americans get more than enough omega-6 fatty acids.

The AHA diet outlined in Chapter 12 (see page 196) provides a healthy balance of omega-3 and omega-6 fatty acids. As recently mentioned, any EFA supplements should be discussed with a healthcare provider before use in an anti-stroke plan. It is important to remember that fish oil pills, which are the most common form of EFA supplement, are also natural blood thinners, which is another reason a stroke patient should ask his doctor about EFA supplements before using them to prevent another stroke. Since fish oil increases the risk of bleeding (in the brain, gastrointestinal tract, etc.), it may amplify the effect of any antithrombotic medication a patient may be taking to prevent stroke (e.g., aspirin, clopidogrel, warfarin, NOACs), putting him at high risk of catastrophic hemorrhage. In addition, people who have had hemorrhagic strokes are advised to avoid fish oil supplements.

ANTIOXIDANTS

Oxidative stress can damage the brain, blood vessels, and heart muscle cells. (See "Antioxidants and Free Radicals" on page 157.) Antioxidants counteract oxidative stress by neutralizing free radicals. While this chapter has discussed both vitamin and mineral antioxidants, the following antioxidants are neither vitamins nor minerals but still play an important role in protecting the body from free radicals and the damage they can inflict.

Alpha-Lipoic Acid

Alpha-lipoic acid (ALA) is a nutrient that is present in the mitochondria of cells, commonly known as the "powerhouses of cells," where it is used in energy production. Well known for its antioxidant powers, ALA can neutralize a variety of free radicals and prevent oxidative stress. This nutrient has also been shown to improve insulin sensitivity, which leads to lower blood sugar levels, in type 2 diabetics. ALA has been studied in small groups of stroke patients, but no large studies have tested if supplements of ALA may be beneficial after stroke, so at this time, it's best to get ALA from the diet. Foods high in ALA include spinach, cow kidney and heart, broccoli, tomatoes, peas, Brussels sprouts, and rice bran.

Anthocyanins

Anthocyanins are chemicals that give red, purple, blue, or black fruits and vegetables their intense coloring. They are also strong antioxidants. Studies have shown that people who eat foods rich in anthocyanins are less likely to have cardiovascular disease. These foods include blackberries, blueberries, cranberries, purple grapes, and plums. Eggplants, sweet potatoes, and red cabbage also contain anthocyanins. There are supplements of anthocyanins available, but it is preferable to acquire these substances from foods, which contain lots of other valuable nutrients—fiber, vitamins, and minerals—necessary for good health.

Cacao, Cocoa, and Chocolate

Chocolate is a mixed blessing. On one hand, it's very addictive due to the high sugar or corn syrup content needed to balance its naturally bitter taste. (More about sugar and its addictive properties in Chapter 11 on page 175. This is an important subject, as any stroke patient or at-risk person should try to eliminate added sugar in his diet, which is associated with weight gain, elevated blood sugar, and general disruption of metabolism.) On the other hand, ground cocoa contains more than a hundred different compounds, including strong anti-oxidant and anti-inflammatory chemicals. Research has shown that cocoa or chocolate intake modestly reduces both systolic and diastolic blood pressures. Other studies have reported that cocoa or chocolate reduces some health factors associated with diabetes. It seems not, however, to lower cholesterol, triglycerides, or blood sugar.

A review of fifteen studies that looked at the association between chocolate intake and stroke found a reduction in stroke risk of 3.5 percent with each increase in chocolate intake of 20 grams, but the benefit was highest with an intake of 45 grams of chocolate a week, which is equivalent to approximately one square of chocolate per day or about one chocolate bar per week.

It is essential to understand that all cocoa-based products are not equally healthy. Cacao powder is made by cold-pressing (relying only on pressure, without the use of heat) unroasted cocoa beans. It contains all the nutrients found in the beans. Cocoa powder is made from raw cacao that has been roasted at a high temperature, reducing its overall nutritional value. Chocolate refers to the confection made by adding cocoa butter, sugar, and other ingredients to cocoa powder. Milk chocolate also includes milk proteins, which further decrease cocoa's benefits. White chocolate has no known health benefits.

If your goal is to improve health with cocoa bean-related products, choose those that contain high amounts of cacao or cocoa and no sugar or corn syrup. A safe sugar substitute, such as monk fruit, unprocessed honey, stevia, or xylitol, may be as a sweetener instead.

For chocolate lovers who would like to enjoy the benefits of cocoa without the sugar issue, there are many recipes for dark chocolate treats that use unprocessed honey, monk fruit, stevia, or xylitol. (See inset on page 171.) For those who would rather buy ready-made chocolate, they should look for products that have a high percentage of cacao and no sugar. For example, ChocZero Ultimate Dark chocolate squares, which are antioxidant rich and sweetened with monk fruit, not sugar. Another example is Lily's Dark Chocolate, which is sweetened with stevia. While dark chocolate may be good for you, it is still high in calories, so no more than one or two square inches of dark chocolate should be eaten in one day.

It is important to note that chocolate can be problematic for some people. Individuals who are allergic to chocolate may develop skin rashes or other allergic symptoms when they eat chocolate. If you have headaches, try reducing your cacao intake. High cacao consumption is associated with migraines. Chocolate is also known to interact with certain drugs. For example, chocolate can increase the risk of bleeding when taken with blood-thinning medications such as warfarin, aspirin, or ibuprofen. A doctor or pharmacist can provide more information about interactions between cacao and drugs.

Coenzyme Q$_{10}$

Coenzyme Q$_{10}$ (CoQ$_{10}$) is a fat-soluble nutrient that can be found in almost every cell of the body, where it plays an important part in producing cellular energy. Also a powerful antioxidant, it is called a coenzyme because it helps enzymes do their job.

In a study of many studies, patients with coronary artery disease who took CoQ$_{10}$ supplements significantly lowered total cholesterol levels and increased good cholesterol levels. CoQ$_{10}$ has also been proposed to relieve the muscle aches that some patients experience with statin drugs, but the results of studies have been mixed. CoQ$_{10}$ has not been significantly studied in relation to stroke. A healthcare provider should advise a patient on whether he should take a CoQ$_{10}$ supplement. A daily dosage of 100 mg may be helpful.

Garlic

Garlic is a common flavoring agent used in cooking a variety of foods and has also been used for centuries for health and medicinal purposes. It is a member of the allium family of plants and is related to onions, shallots, and leeks. Garlic contains a special sulfur compound called allicin, which is responsible for its "garlicky" smell and its healing properties. Allicin is a strong antioxidant and anti-inflammatory compound.

Garlic has all kinds of effects on stroke risk factors. It reduces total cholesterol and bad cholesterol but only slightly increases good cholesterol. It also significantly reduces fasting blood sugar and lowers high blood pressure, both systolic and diastolic.

Although garlic supplements are widely available, many researchers recommend consuming garlic as a food until more scientific studies have been done on garlic supplementation. Thankfully, it can be used many different foods, including salad dressings, vegetables, meats, soups, stews, and sauces.

Melatonin

Melatonin is a hormone that is well known for its role in helping induce sleep. For years people have used supplements of this hormone as a natural sleep aid. It works by adjusting the natural biorhythms, which can be disturbed by a stroke.

As you know, oxidative stress and inflammation increase greatly after a stroke, causing brain damage. Melatonin may hold promise as a neuroprotectant after stroke, as it may combat inflammation and neutralize free radicals, but it has not been studied in large trials of stroke patients. Therefore, at this time, there is no evidence to suggest that melatonin supplements aid in stroke recovery.

Melatonin has been shown to relieve sleep disturbances and depression, which are exceedingly common in stroke patients. Getting better sleep and feeling more motivated will allow a patient to perform better in rehab. Melatonin is produced by the body and cannot be found in foods, but several foods—including pineapples, oranges, bananas, oats, sweet corn, rice, barley, and tomatoes—have been found to boost melatonin production. It may also be taken in supplement form. A typically daily dosage is 0.2 mg to 1 mg, but a patient should discuss supplementation with his doctor before beginning any regimen.

Quercetin

Quercetin belongs to a group of plant pigments called flavonoids, which give fruits and vegetables their colors. Like many flavonoids, quercetin is an antioxidant, anti-inflammatory, anti-clotting substance that slows the aging process. It is found in a number of plants and plant-based foods, including apples, red wine, dark red cherries, berries, tomatoes, broccoli, cabbage, spinach, kale, and citrus fruits.

A dietary study of the intake of flavonoids reported that an elevated intake reduced the incidence of and mortality from cardiovascular disease. An analysis of studies showed that quercetin supplements may significantly reduce both systolic and diastolic blood pressures. It further reported that doses of 500 mg or more had significant effects while lower doses did not. A healthcare provider should be able to advise her patient about quercetin supplements, although a healthy diet of lots of fruits and vegetables should be the main source of quercetin.

Advice for Caregivers

HOMEMADE CHOCOLATE SQUARES

If you are a caregiver for a stroke patient who likes chocolate, here's an easy, inexpensive recipe for making dark chocolate that is far healthier than most of the products sold in stores. Start by buying organic cocoa butter—it comes in chunks, so you will have to estimate the amount for a cup—ground cocoa or cacao, vanilla extract, one of the sweeteners listed below, and raw walnuts at your local health food store or online.

These amounts you will need are as follows:

1 cup cocoa butter

1 cup cocoa or cacao powder

1 teaspoon pure vanilla extract

1 cup unprocessed honey, stevia, monk fruit, or xylitol

1 cup raw unprocessed walnuts

Spray the bottom and sides of an 8 x 8-inch cake pan with vegetable oil. Evenly spread the walnuts along the bottom. Place the cocoa butter in the top of a double boiler over boiling water. Reduce the heat to low and wait for the cocoa butter to completely melt. Add the cocoa powder, sweetener, and vanilla to the mixture and stir until smooth. Taste the mixture and add a little more sweetener if needed. Spread it over the walnuts and refrigerate until firm. Cut or break into approximately sixteen 2-inch squares.

The cocoa in these squares provides beneficial phytochemicals while the walnuts provide omega-3 fatty acids. If your loved one has problems swallowing or chewing, just omit the walnuts until he is better.

Resveratrol

Resveratrol is one of the most popular chemical compounds of the last few years. The chief biologically active component in red wine, this substance is also found in grape juice, blueberries, cranberries, and peanuts, but in far smaller amounts. The resveratrol in red wine comes from the skin of the grapes used to make the wine.

A strong antioxidant, resveratrol helps prevent blood clots and damage to blood vessels, and reduces bad cholesterol. While it sounds like it would be perfect in helping to prevent strokes and heart attacks, the scientific evidence is not yet compelling enough to suggest taking resveratrol supplements.

One glass of red wine each day for a woman and two for a man would supply a good amount of resveratrol. More alcohol than that is not recommended. People who have experienced hemorrhagic strokes are advised to avoid alcohol altogether, as it is associated with increased rates of brain bleeds. Of course, someone who does not normally drink alcohol but is hoping to prevent a stroke should not start drinking wine simply to do so. There are other ways to lower stroke risk. Grape juice may not be an appropriate choice either, as it contains concentrated amounts of fructose without the fiber to slow the absorption of sugar, causing blood sugar to go up quickly. A healthy nonalcoholic option would be to eat red or purple grapes or the other foods mentioned earlier.

Turmeric (Curcumin)

Turmeric, also known as the "golden spice," is derived from the root of a plant that has been used for centuries in East Asian, South Asian, and Middle Eastern cooking—curries, for example—but also in Indian and Chinese medicine. After the root has been boiled and dried, it is ground into a powder, becoming the bright orange-colored spice known as turmeric. Turmeric does not dissolve in water but is soluble in fat and oil, so consuming it with olive oil may aid in the body's absorption of this substance. A small amount of black pepper may also help.

While turmeric contains many health-promoting substances, the key active component of this spice is a compound called curcumin, which has strong antioxidant, anti-inflammatory, and anti-tumor effects. Curcumin is currently being studied for both prevention and treatment of type 2 diabetes, heart disease, brain disorders, and different cancers. Data from various studies suggest that curcumin is well-tolerated and safe for humans.

Studies in animals suggest that turmeric may reduce the risk of stroke and improve the outcome after a stroke, but there is not enough evidence yet to recommend turmeric supplements for stroke patients. Although more convincing research is needed, consuming more meals that include turmeric, such as curries, stews, or rice dishes, is a worthwhile choice.

CONCLUSION

With all this information in hand, a stroke patient and his healthcare provider should be able to create a nutritional plan that supports better health and decreases his risk of another stroke. You may think a patient could simply take a multivitamin to provide all the nutrients he needs to prevent a stroke, eliminating the need to consider his diet. If so, think again. According to research, multivitamins probably do not reduce the risk of stroke. Eating a healthy diet, on the other hand, can lower stroke risk considerably. A healthcare provider may recommend certain supplements but food should provide the first line of defense.

Chapters 11, 12, and 13 discuss an anti-stroke diet and offer guidance in selecting more fruits and vegetables, whole grains, lean meat and poultry, fish, unprocessed nuts, and low-fat milk and cheese, and in eating less red meat, processed meat, saturated fat, sugar, and white flour. Choosing the right foods and avoiding bad foods can greatly reduce a person's chance of having a stroke and help him heal if he has already had one. As the saying goes, let food be thy medicine.

11

$\mathscr{F}$oods to Avoid

W hen it comes to good health, diet matters. We are truly reflections of what we eat. If we eat foods that are little better than garbage, we will feel like garbage. To put it another way, the human body is like a computer. If you enter bad data into a computer, you cannot expect it to come up with accurate output. Likewise, if you continually feed yourself the wrong foods, you should not be surprised when your body fails to work properly.

In recent years, it has become more and more clear that our most common chronic diseases—including stroke—are largely caused by poor lifestyle choices, including what we eat. Having a stroke is a high price to pay for indulging in fast food, processed food, sugary beverages, and salty or sugary snacks. To prevent a first stroke or a future stroke, a person should change what he eats on a daily basis so that his diet provides the nutrients his body needs to preserve, protect, and heal blood vessels and brain cells. He should also avoid including foods in his diet that can clog his arteries, spike his blood glucose levels, or otherwise contribute to having a stroke.

The American Heart Association (AHA) diet (see page 196) was devised by many medical and nutritional experts. The purpose of the AHA diet is to reduce risk factors for heart disease and stroke. It is meant to lower high blood pressure, regulate blood sugar, encourage weight loss, and greatly improve overall nutrition. This simple diet plan allows grocery shopping to go more quickly and easily. It also provides foods that can make preventing a first stroke or avoiding a second stroke a delicious endeavor.

Since everyone's taste is different, it's important to remember that there are a number of other anti-stroke diets to consider, including the Mediterranean diet, the DASH diet (Dietary Approaches to Stop Hypertension), and the MIND diet (Mediterranean-DASH Intervention for Neurodegenerative Delay). The overall idea with any of these diet plans is to eat less saturated and trans fats, salt (sodium), sugar, and red meat; and to eat more fruits and vegetables, whole grains, fish and poultry, unprocessed nuts and seeds, legumes, and dairy. (See page 291 of the Resources for more information on these diets.)

This chapter discusses the "bad," or unhealthy, dietary components to avoid or eat as infrequently as possible and lists common foods that contribute to stroke risk. Chapter 12 presents the other half of the issue of diet: the foods to put on your plate—foods like fruits, vegetables, whole grains, and so on. Finally, Chapter 13 shows you how to put the anti-stroke diet into action.

Advice for Caregivers
LEARNING ABOUT THE ANTI-STROKE DIET

If your loved one has had a stroke and you are helping him with his grocery shopping, you could take it upon yourself to learn about the anti-stroke diet and then teach him how to eat to avoid another stroke. If you, too, begin to change your diet for the better, you may encourage him to stick to this lifestyle choice. Both of you could become healthier together!

INGREDIENTS TO AVOID OR LIMIT

A "bad" ingredient is one that disrupts normal metabolism—which refers both to the body's ability to break down food for energy and manufacture substances that are necessary for life—and over time makes your organs function poorly or even shut down. These ingredients could be considered "anti-nutrients," as they are essentially the opposite of the healthy nutrients discussed in the previous chapter. By learning about common anti-nutrients, a stroke patient can better understand which foods to avoid or limit in order to prevent a second stroke, and an at-risk individual will know how to reduce his risk of experiencing a first stroke.

Saturated Fat

The typical American diet contains lots of saturated fat. Saturated fat is found primarily in animal products, including whole milk, cheese, and fatty meats—beef, veal, lamb, pork, and ham. The marbling you see in beef and pork, in fact, is composed of saturated fat. Some vegetable products—including processed coconut oil, palm kernel oil, and solid vegetable shortening—are also high in saturated fat. Saturated fat is generally solid at room temperature.

Not all saturated fats are created equal, and not all saturated fats are bad for you. Foods are not simply a collection of components, such as fat and protein, but a complex matrix that can have a variety of effects on health. Different foods can have different effects on hunger, feelings of fullness, sugar metabolism, hormone responses, fat production, gut bacteria, and the body's metabolic rate. This area of research is rapidly evolving, but from what we know, it seems that saturated fat from meat is associated with a higher risk of cardiovascular disease while saturated fat from dairy is associated with a lower risk of cardiovascular disease.

A collection of twenty-nine studies that included nearly one million participants showed that total dairy and milk consumption were not associated with death, heart disease, or cardiovascular disease, and suggested that fermented dairy products (e.g., cheese, yogurt) were associated with a lower risk of death from cardiovascular disease. In fact, the consumption of cheese alone—the dairy product with the highest amount of dairy fat—was associated with lower risks of both heart disease and stroke.

Studies have also found that consuming dairy alters body composition, reducing body fat and increasing muscle mass. Contrary to decades of popular belief, whole-fat dairy does not increase the risk of weight gain, type 2 diabetes, or cardiovascular disease. A collection of thirty-seven randomized trials that included 184,802 participants showed that dairy consumption did not affect body mass index but instead led to a reduction in fat and an increase in lean body mass.

In the Malmö Diet and Cancer Cohort study, which followed nearly 27,000 participants over fourteen years, low-fat dairy consumption was associated with a higher risk of type 2 diabetes, whereas whole-fat dairy consumption was associated with a lower risk.

So, why is whole-fat dairy good for you while fatty meat is not, despite the fact that both foods contain large amounts of saturated fat? It could be because whole-fat dairy products contain more short-chain and medium-chain fatty acids than meat, which contains a higher proportion of long-chain fatty acids. Short- and medium-chain fatty acids may have beneficial effects on metabolism, weight, and the bacteria in the intestines, also known as the gut microbiome. In addition, probiotics found in fermented dairy products, such as yogurt and kefir, may also positively impact the gut microbiome. In fact, a summary of fifteen trials showed that probiotics played a role in weight loss and body fat reduction in overweight individuals.

The fact is that some saturated fats are considered unhealthy because they can raise LDL cholesterol (the "bad" kind of cholesterol), placing a person at a higher risk of both heart disease and stroke. As saturated fat can contribute to plaque formation, which can compromise circulation and impede blood flow to the heart and brain, it is a factor that should not be ignored in regard to stroke prevention, even if some foods with saturated fat may not be as unhealthy as we have been told in the past.

How Much Saturated Fat Is Safe to Eat?

The American Heart Association recommends that no more than 5 to 6 percent of total daily calories come from saturated fat. So, if you eat roughly 2,000 calories per day, your saturated fat calories should not exceed 140 calories, or 11 to 13 grams. In the average diet, which is full of fast food and processed foods, grams of fat add up in a hurry along with calories. For example, 8 ounces of 80 percent ground beef contains approximately 18 grams of saturated fat and 580 calories per serving; a large pork chop contains approximately 7 grams of saturated fat and 320 calories; and a small vanilla milkshake from Dairy Queen contains approximately 14 grams of saturated fat and 520 calories.

Clearly, it's important to be aware of the amount of saturated fat found in the foods you eat. So, when buying packaged foods, always check the "Nutrition Facts" label, which states how much saturated fat and total fat are provided by each serving of a product. (See page 191 for information on reading food labels.)

TRANS FAT

A small amount of trans fat occurs naturally in meat and dairy products, but most of the trans fats in the food supply is from the process of creating partially hydrogenated vegetable fat. Partially hydrogenated fat was manufactured in factories by adding hydrogen to liquid unsaturated fat in order to make it solid. It was used by food companies to improve shelf life and keep flavors stable, and could be found in countless processed foods, including frozen pizza, doughnuts, cakes, pie crusts, biscuits, cookies, crackers, margarine, and other spreads.

Researchers found that trans fat behaves much like saturated fat in the body but is even more damaging to an individual's health. Like saturated fat, trans fat raises levels of harmful LDL cholesterol. In addition, it lowers levels of healthy HDL cholesterol. These reactions increase the risks of coronary heart disease, stroke, type 2 diabetes, Alzheimer's, and cancer. After trans fats had been linked to these health conditions, a law was passed in the United States that led manufacturers that use trans fats to replace them with healthier options.

No amount of trans fat is considered a safe amount to consume. As explained, at this time there should be no artificial trans fats in the food supply, but be sure to check all Nutrition Facts labels when you purchase packaged foods just to be sure. Be aware, however, that manufacturers are required to list the amount of trans fats in a product only if it amounts to 0.5 grams or more per serving. In other words, a label can list 0 trans fat content even if a small amount is present. In addition, be sure to read the ingredients of a product to see if any partially hydrogenated fat is included—a sure sign the product contains trans fats.

Sodium (Salt)

High blood pressure, or hypertension, accounts for more than 50 percent of all strokes. As such, it is the single most important stroke risk factor. It is also an incredibly common stroke risk factor, as approximately 46 percent of Americans have high blood pressure. If a stroke patient has high blood pressure, his healthcare provider will discuss with him the importance of reducing salt (sodium) in his diet. Salt increases blood volume, thereby increasing blood pressure.

Anyone interested in reducing salt intake should begin by using less salt (or no salt at all) when cooking and at the dinner table. One way to do so would be to use a table salt with less sodium, such as Morton's Lite Salt, which has half the sodium content of regular salt (the sodium is partly replaced with potassium). Another way to cut down on sodium intake would be to use additional spices or herbs instead of salt.

Be aware, though, that about 75 percent of the sodium in the average American diet comes from restaurant food and packaged foods. For example, a single dinner at a Chinese restaurant may come with about 2,400 mg of sodium or more. So, any person who would like to control his sodium intake will have to avoid many restaurant meals and check the Nutrition Facts label on every food he is interested in purchasing. (A restaurant may be able to prepare certain meals with little to no salt if such a request is made.)

Advice for Caregivers
REDUCING DIETARY SALT

While your loved one is recovering from his stroke, whether in a hospital, rehabilitation facility, or his home, you can help him opt for meals that are low in sodium. (Your loved one's doctor may have already ordered a low-sodium diet to help control his high blood pressure.) Some foods that are extremely high in sodium include canned soups and processed meat. You could ask a registered dietitian to explain to both your loved one and you which foods are high in sodium. If a dietitian visits your loved one, take notes on the information she presents. You could also ask her if there is a hand-out that details high-sodium foods. Knowing more about the dangers of too much salt, you can steer your loved one away from foods like sausage, bacon, fries, chips, and pretzels, and towards healthier options with less sodium.

How Much Salt Is Safe to Eat?

The American Heart Association recommends limiting sodium to less than 2,300 milligrams of sodium per day—about one teaspoon—and ideally no more than 1,500 milligrams each day. Reducing blood pressure to normal levels is important in preventing a stroke. Remember that high blood pressure is the leading preventable cause of stroke.

Clearly, it's important to be aware of foods that are most likely to provide large amounts of sodium. Table 11.1 states the sodium count for a number of common foods.

TABLE 11.1. SODIUM CONTENT OF COMMON FOODS

Food	Sodium Per Serving
1 slice bacon	137 mg
1 slice ham	360 mg
1 ounce breakfast sausage	302 mg
1 ounce potato chips	175–185 mg
1 ounce pretzels	359 mg
1 slice pepperoni pizza	400 mg
1 ounce (39 nuts) dry-roasted peanuts, salted	230 mg
1 tablespoon soy sauce	511–1,000 mg
1 veggie burger	398 mg
1/2 cup tomato sauce	642 mg
1 cup vegetable juice	500 mg
1 slice whole wheat bread	240–400 mg
1 bowl cereal	170–300 mg
2 tablespoons reduced-fat Italian salad dressing	260 mg
1/2 cup cottage cheese	270 mg

By looking at Table 11.1, it is easy to see some of the biggest sodium offenders. The sodium content of soy sauce, for example, varies greatly by brand and may reach 1,000 mg per tablespoon. In the case of tomato sauce or vegetable juice, it should be easy to find low-sodium options, but it's important to read the Nutrition Facts label to determine the exact sodium amount of any product.

It is important to note that many foods with significant amounts of sodium are unhealthy for other reasons, too. Bacon, for instance, has lots of saturated fat and preservatives. Luncheon meats, sausage, and hot dogs contain similar anti-nutrients and are associated with increased stroke risk. Potato chips are made with vegetable oil that has been used over and over again, creating toxins. So, how do you avoid these anti-nutrients? In general, the more you stay away from processed foods, the healthier you will be.

Sugar

Sugar seems to be everywhere in the average diet, and as you may be aware, it poses a significant danger to health. Evidence is growing that this simple ingredient, which can appear under many different names, is a chief culprit in the development of many of the disorders that plague modern society and that can contribute to stroke.

In order to better understand this ingredient, you need to learn about the four basic types of sugar. At least one type of sugar is bound to be contained in many of the food products you buy. (To see all of sugar's many names, consult inset on page 183.) The four types of sugar are similar in chemical structure, but each is ultimately unique.

Glucose is the sugar that circulates in the blood and provides the body with energy. It is the sugar that is elevated in the blood of diabetics. Lactose, or "milk sugar," is naturally found in milk. The Nutrition Facts label of an average carton of whole milk list 12 grams of sugar per cup. That sugar is lactose. Generally, this type of sugar does not cause health problems unless the person consuming it is lactose intolerant.

Fructose, or "fruit sugar," is found naturally in fruits and vegetables. The fiber in fruits and vegetables helps slow the body's absorption of fructose so it doesn't lead to spikes in blood sugar. When fruit is turned into juice, the fiber is removed, and so drinking juice can lead to blood sugar spikes. Turning whole fruits and vegetables into smoothies, however, retains the healthy fiber, making smoothies a better choice when it comes to blood sugar levels. Of course, fructose is also found in high-fructose corn syrup, which is an ingredient to avoid completely.

SUGAR BY ANY OTHER NAME

Sugar may be found in the ingredients lists of packaged foods under many different names. Some products include a number of these names on a single label. Names for sugar include agave, cane juice, corn syrup, dextrose, fruit juice concentrate, maltose, and many others.

The "sugars" entry on a Nutrition Facts label provides the total sugar content of a product. The amount of "added sugars," which refer to the sugars added to a product, may also be listed on a product's label.

Sucrose, commonly referred to as table sugar, is found naturally in some fruits, but most dietary sucrose comes from granulated sugar, which is extracted from sugar cane or beets.

Sugar Addiction

Humans are born with a preference for things that taste sweet. This preference is evident even in the womb, as studies suggest unborn babies swallow more amniotic fluid when it is sweet rather than bitter or sour. This preference is especially helpful after birth, as it encourages a baby to drink breast milk or formula, both of which contain sugar. After a child has been weaned, however, consumption of too many sugar-laden foods and beverages can lead to sugar addiction.

Food manufacturers count on this addiction, adding sugar in one form or another to almost everything. Approximately 75 percent of packaged foods in the United States contain added sugar. Regular soft drinks, fruit drinks, energy drinks, and sports drinks are all full of sugar or high-fructose corn syrup. Sugary treats have become a crucial part of every celebration, from birthdays to weddings to funerals. And for many people, the meal isn't complete until a sugary dessert is eaten.

So, can you really become "addicted" to sugar? According to scientific research there is such a thing as sugar addiction, and most

Americans are hooked. Withdrawal effects are similar to those of taking away drugs from drug abusers: binging, withdrawal, depression, and craving.

As a person consumes more and more sugar, it takes a toll on his body. If the amount of glucose is greater than what his cells need, the excess is stored as fat. This is why sugar consumption is a major contributor to obesity. Sugar has also been shown to contribute to the development of cardiovascular disease, fatty liver disease, hypertension, type 2 diabetes, and kidney disease.

As dangerous as excessive table sugar is to health, high-fructose corn syrup appears to be even more harmful. High-fructose corn syrup first became available in 1967, and its consumption took off like a rocket. Consumers loved it, probably because fructose is 1.7 times sweeter than sucrose. Food manufacturers loved it because it was cheaper than table sugar and enhanced the taste and shelf life of their products. Soon it was being used to sweeten not only beverages—sodas, fruit drinks, and soft drinks—but also candies, breads, cereals, breakfast bars, yogurt, and much more.

Advice for Caregivers
REDUCING SUGAR CONSUMPTION

If you are caring for a stroke patient who is a "sugar-holic"—and perhaps diabetic or prediabetic—you will want to suggest to him that he reduce his sweets slowly. If he suddenly goes without sugar, he may feel crummy and experience intense cravings for anything sweet.

If your loved one has always guzzled lots of soda, suggest that he cut back to one soda a day for a few days, and then to half a soda, and so on, until he no longer drinks soda at all. Suggest to his friends that they not bring candy or sweet desserts to him when they visit. Tell him to go easy on hospital desserts and suggest he opt for fruit without added sugar instead. He may be grumpy about these changes, but you will be doing him a huge favor that will help him once he leaves the hospital or rehab and is on his own. Support him by resisting sweet beverages and foods yourself. In the end, you will feel better too and be healthier!

Before long, researchers began to suspect that this new sweetener brought with it real problems. Fructose fails to stimulate the production of insulin and leptin, two hormones that normally help regulate food consumption and body weight, and which are triggered by regular sugar. Thus, fructose is believed to play a major role in the obesity epidemic, which has led to increases in hypertension, type 2 diabetes, and other major health problems. Moreover, a high intake of fructose can lead to fatty liver disease.

How Much Sugar Is Safe to Eat?

The American Heart Association recommends that women consume no more than 6 teaspoons of sugar each day, while men should consume no more than 9 teaspoons. Unfortunately, it is all too easy to exceed these amounts with just one or two sweetened foods or beverages. For example, one slice of Betty Crocker Extra Moist Yellow Cake (without icing) contains almost 5 teaspoons of sugar from table sugar and corn syrup. In addition, twelve ounces of Coke contain almost 10 teaspoons of sugar in the form of high-fructose corn syrup; one cup of Fruit Loops contains 3 teaspoons of table sugar; half a cup of Del Monte Fruit Cocktail in heavy syrup contains over 5 teaspoons of sugar in the form of high-fructose corn syrup, corn syrup, and table sugar; two tablespoons of Kraft Catalina Salad Dressing contain 2 teaspoons of table sugar; two tablespoons of Heinz Ketchup contain 2 teaspoons of sugar from high-fructose corn syrup and corn syrup; and one cup of Ragu Old World Style Traditional Spaghetti Sauce contains 2 teaspoons of table sugar.

When it comes to sugar consumption, the best advice is to avoid high-fructose corn syrup altogether and consume as little other added sugars as possible, with the goal being zero. Eating sugary foods creates the desire for more sugary foods, feeding the addiction. If a stroke survivor is used to having a lot of sugar-laden foods in his diet, however, he should not try to go cold turkey and eliminate all added sugar at once. Doing so may cause him to experience anxiety, shakiness, or intense cravings. He should slowly decrease the amount of sugar in recipes, stop buying sugary foods, and avoid soda or other drinks that contain sugar. His body will thank him.

Artificial Sweeteners

Some people think that if sugar is harmful, it makes sense to choose foods and beverages prepared with artificial sweeteners. After all, the average can of soda packs about 150 calories, nearly all of them from sugar or corn syrup, while the same amount of diet soda delivers zero calories and therefore shouldn't contribute to weight gain and all its complications. Unfortunately, studies show that artificial sweeteners have their own adverse effects.

First, it may surprise you to learn that consumers who use artificial sweeteners are at an increased risk of excessive weight gain, metabolic syndrome, type 2 diabetes, high blood pressure, and cardiovascular disease, including stroke. Moreover, a high consumption of artificially sweetened soft drinks is associated with a higher risk of dementia.

Various explanations have been offered for some of the problems caused by these additives. For instance, non-nutritive (diet) sweeteners may change the way that people taste food by overstimulating the sugar receptors. This may lead people to crave sweetness and eat only intensely sweet high-calorie foods, while avoiding healthy "unsweet" foods like vegetables. Even fruit may not be sweet enough for people used to artificially sweetened fare. In addition, some people think that because they're saving calories by drinking diet beverages, they are free to eat high-calorie, high-sugar food, such as cake, ice cream, or cookies.

Several studies have also shown that the artificial sweeteners saccharin, sucralose, and aspartame cause problems by altering healthy gut bacteria. In one study, healthy volunteers consumed saccharin for one week. They quickly developed altered intestinal bacteria and poorer glucose tolerance.

The bottom line is that artificial sweeteners such as aspartame (Equal, NutraSweet, and Natra Taste Blue), saccharin (Sweet 'N Low), and sucralose (Splenda) should be avoided. Diet drinks can be used for a short time as a replacement for sugar-sweetened beverages, but the goal should be to stop drinking soda altogether. The next chapter discusses four alternative sweeteners that appear to be safe: stevia, monk fruit, xylitol, and unprocessed honey. But even then, sweeteners should be used sparingly in order to control addiction to anything sweet.

Alcohol

As discussed in Chapter 2, too much alcohol is a risk factor for stroke. Small to moderate amounts of alcohol appear to be protective against cardiovascular disease, including ischemic strokes, but not hemorrhagic strokes, while heavy amounts increase the risk of both ischemic and hemorrhagic strokes. Stroke patients and at-risk individuals would do well to monitor their alcohol use closely and reduce it if necessary. If one has a history of alcoholism or binge drinking, it's best to avoid alcohol altogether.

FOODS TO AVOID OR LIMIT

Now that we have explored the unhealthiest components of our foods, let's look at the foods and beverages that are most detrimental to both overall health and cardiovascular diseases, including stroke. As you may have guessed, these foods and beverages contain one or more harmful components. They are also commonly found in the average diet.

Sweet Beverages

Greater consumption of sugar-sweetened beverages is associated with a greater risk of stroke. Most commercial beverages are a minefield of harmful ingredients. Soft drinks, energy drinks, and sports beverages are almost all loaded with sugar, corn syrup, or artificial sweeteners. Considering that both sugar and artificial sweeteners increase a person's appetite for more sweet foods, it's no wonder many Americans have an obesity problem. And, as you know, obesity is a risk factor for stroke and other disorders.

Colas and a number of other beverages contain caffeine, which can cause a short but dramatic rise in blood pressure—another stroke risk factor. Colas also contain phosphoric acid, which binds calcium, magnesium, and zinc in your intestine making them unusable by the body. In addition, the caramel color in cola beverages can lead to formation of harmful chemicals that are known to contribute to the hardening of your arteries, heart disease, kidney disease, and Alzheimer's disease.

How Many Sweet Beverages Are Safe to Drink?

The AHA recommends consuming less than one serving of sweet beverages each day. Ideally, it's best to avoid sweetened beverages altogether. Even one sugary drink a day can feed a sugar addiction and leave a person wanting more sweet treats.

Good beverage choices include milk; black, green, or herbal tea; coffee; and cocoa—preferably without sugar or heavy cream. (The next chapter discusses the positive effects of tea, coffee, and cocoa, which can actually help protect against stroke.) The best choice is, of course, a refreshing glass of water, which can be flavored with a squeeze of lemon or lime juice. If you feel the need to add a little sweetener to certain beverages, keep it light and replace refined sugar with a healthier option. It is advisable, however, to try to get used to drinking beverages that have little or no sweetener of any kind. Believe it or not, you can re-educate your taste buds to appreciate drinks that are unsweetened.

Red Meat

Red meat—beef, pork, and lamb—contains significant amounts of beneficial nutrients: protein, iron, zinc, and B vitamins, especially vitamin B_{12}. Americans consume too much red meat, though, which is high in saturated fat, cholesterol, and calories, increasing heart disease and stroke risks. The more red meat and processed meats a person eats, the higher his stroke risk becomes. One study reported that participants who substituted poultry for one serving of red meat lowered their risk of stroke. A high intake of red meat has also been linked to cancer, kidney failure, type 2 diabetes, and even Alzheimer's disease. Processed meats are even more destructive.

How Much Red Meat Is Safe to Eat?

The AHA recommends limiting red meat consumption. The Mediterranean diet recommends limiting red and processed meats to less than one serving per day. When choosing red meat, always opt for the leanest cuts with very little visible fat or marbling. Trim off as much fat as you can. Ground beef should be 93 percent lean. Pork or beef that has "loin" or "round" in its name is usually the leanest choice.

Beef labeled "prime" usually has more fat. (See Table 11.2. Saturated Fat in Three Ounces of Red Meat below.)

If a stroke survivor happens to be a big meat eater, he should reduce the number of times he eats red meat in a week while also decreasing the serving size. Chicken or fish, which should be cooked without frying, could be eaten instead of red meat. Alternatively, a plant-based meal can be an inexpensive and delicious low- or no-fat option that's packed with nutrients. If he wants to splurge on a steak, he should order the smallest, leanest cut available, or cut a large portion in half and share it with a loved one. The momentary pleasure of having a huge, fatty steak is not worth increasing the risk of having another stroke.

TABLE 11.2. SATURATED FAT IN THREE OUNCES OF RED MEAT

Meat	Total Fat	Saturated Fat	Calories
Ground beef (70% lean)	24 g	9 g	279
Ground beef (93% lean)	6 g	2 g	148
Boneless prime rib	15 g	6 g	226
Round steak	3 g	2 g	155
Sirloin steak	12 g	3 g	207
Baked boneless ham	14 g	5 g	207
Pork chop	7 g	3 g	118
Lamb chop	18 g	8 g	112

Processed Food

Any food that has been purposely changed in some way before its consumption is considered processed food. If it seems like this word can be applied to a wide range of foods—some healthy and some harmful—it can. Minimally processed foods include bagged salads, while items such as frozen fruits or vegetables, canned tomatoes, or canned tuna may be considered slightly more processed. Further processed foods include jarred pasta sauces, salad dressings, and other foods that contain additives to enhance flavor and texture. Heavily processed foods include crackers, deli meats, and frozen pizza.

Most food that is minimally processed is not harmful; in fact, much of it makes it easier for us to benefit from foods like salads, fruits, and vegetables. But as foods get more processed—farther from their natural state—healthy nutrients are stripped out, and unwholesome ingredients like salt, sugar, corn syrup, and preservatives are added.

Most refined foods are created for longer shelf life; to look, smell, and taste good; and to be easy to prepare—or to require no preparation at all. In some cases, refined foods may be entirely composed of refined products with little to no nutritional benefit. To compensate, a company may add back certain nutrients to make the food seem more like a "real food." These are the foods that are truly damaging to your health. They provide few nutrients to nourish and protect your body, and are packed with harmful ingredients like salt, sugar, and food coloring.

Advice for Caregivers
SERVING A BETTER BREAKFAST

While your loved one is still in the hospital or rehabilitation facility, help him make healthy breakfast choices. Breakfast foods such as pop tarts, pancakes, pastries, donuts, and sweet rolls are high in processed flour, bad fats, and sugar, and should be avoided. He should also skip the sugary cereals that are designed to appeal to children—Cocoa Puffs, Fruit Loops, Captain Crunch, and so on. They are not good for stroke patients and not good for kids either. A better option would be a whole grain cereal with little to no added sugar or oatmeal. In fact, several studies have shown that oatmeal reduces risk of stroke. In a study that looked at the breakfast habits of over 55,000 individuals over 13.4 years, replacing just one serving a week of white bread or eggs with oatmeal was shown to reduce the risk of stroke.

How Much Processed Food Is Safe to Eat?

Although fresh unprocessed food is always best, minimally processed options such as prewashed greens or frozen veggies are safe to eat and should be increased in everyone's diets. More processed foods like canned tomatoes should be used only in moderation and chosen with care to avoid added salt, sugar, and artificial additives. Organic brands should be purchased whenever possible, as they normally contain better ingredients. Highly processed foods, which are not only void of nutrients but also packed with ingredients that can actually impair health and lead to disorders that are associated with stroke, should be completely avoided.

An example of a very common processed food is a refined grain, such as white flour and white flour products, refined cereal, white rice, or white pasta. The government requires that some of these foods, which have been stripped of their nutrition in the refining process, be enriched with niacin (vitamin B_3), iron, thiamin (vitamin B_1), riboflavin (vitamins B_2), and folic acid. These nutrients are just a few of the substances destroyed during processing. For example, when wheat kernels are processed into white flour, the fiber and nutrient-rich germ are lost, leaving just starch. When eaten, this starch converts to glucose and quickly raises blood sugar levels, as there is no fiber to slow down absorption.

The act of enriching food is like a thief who robs $100 from you and then feels a little guilty and gives you back $10—you're still out $90! You will know if a product has been processed by reading the ingredients list on the package or simply by its name. For example, processed flour may be called "white flour," "enriched white flour," or even "unbleached white flour" (bleached or unbleached, though, it's still white flour); and thiamin, riboflavin, or other enriching nutrients may be listed towards the end of the ingredients list.

Foods and beverages that have unfamiliar chemicals in their ingredients lists should also be avoided. If you cannot pronounce it, don't buy it. If an ingredients list is long, forget the food. Look for whole foods instead.

READING FOOD LABELS

Packaged foods typically come with Nutrition Facts labels and ingredients lists, which allow consumers to make informed decisions when shopping for food. If you are the caregiver of a stroke patient and will be doing his grocery shopping after he returns home, you will need to be able to read all the labels on any packaged foods you buy for him. Once he is able to go to the grocery store for himself, you can show him what you have learned before he does so.

Nutrition Facts

Figure 11.1 (below) is an example of a Nutrition Facts label. As you can see, the label first states the "serving size"—in this case, one cake. Always compare the manufacturer's serving size with what you are actually eating. Most Nutrition Facts labels underestimate what most people eat, and if you consume more than one cake, you'll be getting larger helpings of both the nutrients and the "anti-nutrients" contained in this food.

Below the serving size is the number of "calories" (150) found in one serving and the "calories from fat" (41). The section below this

Nutrition Facts

Serving Size 1 cake (42.5 g)

Amount Per Serving

Calories 150	Calories from Fat 41

	% Daily Value
Total Fat 4.5g	**7%**
Saturated Fat 2.5g	**13%**
Trans Fat 0.0g	
Cholesterol 20g	**7%**
Sodium 220g	**9%**
Total Carbohydrate 27g	**9%**
Sugars 18.0g	
Protein 1.0g	

Vitamin A 0%	•	Vitamin C 0%
Calcium 0%	•	Iron 6%

*Percent Daily Values are based on a 2,000 calorie diet.

Figure 11.1. Nutrition Facts Label

focuses on the fats found in each cake, including "total fat" (4.5 g), "saturated fat" (2.5 g), and "trans fat" (0.0 g). The information stated under "% daily value" tells you this product provides 7 percent of total daily fat intake based on a 2,000-calorie diet. When a packaged food contains polyunsaturated and monounsaturated fats—which are healthier than saturated fats—it will state these counts as well. (This example includes no "good" fats, a sign that the food is not a particularly healthy one.)

Below the section on fats, you'll find "cholesterol" (20 mg), "sodium" (220 mg), and "total carbohydrates" (27 g). Under total carbohydrates, you'll see "sugar" (18 g). There are 4 grams of sugar in 1 teaspoon, so this product contains 4.5 teaspoons of sugar. On some products, like milk and fruit, the amount of sugar listed may be misleading, as these products contain natural sugar—lactose or fructose. This is why it's so important to read the list of ingredients, as it will help you understand the source of the sugar. Packages are required to list "added sugars" so consumers can understand how much sugar that is not naturally present in particular ingredients has been added to a product containing those ingredients.

On many products, such as whole grain bread or brown rice, "fiber" may be listed under "total carbohydrates." But like many unhealthy foods, this snack cake contains no fiber at all. This Nutrition Facts label ends by listing "protein" (only 1 g), no vitamins, and almost no minerals (iron 6%). It should be no surprise that this food product provides no micronutrients except a trace amount of iron, which comes from the enriched white flour.

Ingredients

Figure 11.2 (see page 194) is an example of an Ingredients List of a food product. The considerable number of ingredients listed should act as a warning that this food product is likely unhealthy. Healthy foods usually contain only a few minimally processed ingredients, while junk foods tend to be manufactured from a long list of components, including several that you would never find in an actual kitchen.

Be aware that ingredients are listed in order of content. In other words, the first ingredient listed is also the ingredient of which there is the highest amount. On this label, flour and sugar are the first ingredients stated, meaning that this food is made largely of refined flour and refined sugar, two nutritionally bankrupt foods.

The flour used to make this product is bleached and refined, with four vitamins and iron (ferrous sulfate) added to make up partially for all the good nutrients that were discarded during processing. Four different types of sugar are listed—sugar, corn syrup, high fructose corn syrup, and dextrose. The names may be different, but as you recall from the discussion on page 183, they are all sugar. Next, the label lists partially hydrogenated vegetable shortening, which means that the cake contains harmful trans fats, although the Nutrition Facts label lists none. (Remember, manufacturers don't have to list this ingredient unless there's at least 0.5 grams per serving.)

INGREDIENTS: ENRICHED BLEACHED WHEAT FLOUR [FLOUR, FERROUS SULFATE, "B" VITAMINS (NIACIN, THIAMINE, MONO-NITRATE (B1), RIBOFLAVIN (B2), FOLIC ACID)], SUGAR, CORN SYRUP, WATER, HIGH FRUCTOSE CORN SYRUP, PARTIALLY HYDROGENATED VEGETABLE SHORTENING (CONTAINS ONE OR MORE OF: SOYBEAN, CANOLA OR PALM OIL), DEXTROSE, WHOLE EGGS. CONTAINS 2% OR LESS OF: MODIFIED CORN-STARCH, CELLULOSE GUM, WHEY, LEAVENINGS (SODIUM ACID PYROPHOSPHATE, BAKING SODA, MONOCALCIUM PHOSPHATE), SALT, CORNSTARCH, CORN FLOUR, CORN DEXTRINS, MONO AND DIGLYCERIDES, POLYSORBATE 60, SOY LECITHIN, NATU-RAL AND ARTIFICIAL FLAVORS, SOY PROTEIN ISOLATE, SODIUM STEAROYL LACTYLATE, SODIUM AND CALCIUM CASEINATE, CAL-CIUM SULFATE, SORBIC ACID (TO RETAIN FRESHNESS), COLOR ADDED (YELLOW 5, RED 40). MAY CONTAIN PEANUTS OR TRACES OF PEANUTS.

Figure 11.2.
Ingredients List

The rest of the ingredients are a mystery unless you are a food scientist—polysorbate 60, sodium stearoyl lactylate, and calcium caseinate, for instance. The list ends with two artificial food dyes made from petroleum byproducts—Yellow 5 and Red 40. The use of artificial food coloring in a product almost always means the product lacks many beneficial nutrients.

Although reading food labels may seem a little complicated and time-consuming at first, as you examine more and more products, you will quickly increase your ability to tell good foods from bad ones. Knowledge is power.

CONCLUSION

The task of overhauling your diet or the diet of a loved one may feel overwhelming. And make no mistake, it is not easy. But these changes do not have to be made all in one day. Menus and meals can transform gradually. If you are a stroke survivor, these changes can start in the hospital when you are asked to choose foods for your three meals.

The skill to read food product labels and examine the items in your pantry and refrigerator is invaluable when trying to adopt a new way of eating. Once you know what you are actually eating, you can finish off the questionable food products and make a point of not purchasing them again, or better yet, you can simply give away the foods that don't meet your new standards. If your kitchen starts to seem a little empty, don't worry. The next two chapters will guide you towards the healthy foods that *do* belong on your plate—those that can improve your overall health and prevent a first stroke or a second one.

12

Foods to Eat

N ow that you know about the healthy components of many foods—fiber, protein, vitamins, minerals, essential fatty acids, and phytochemicals—and about the foods that should be avoided or limited in order to prevent a stroke from occurring, we can finally get to the fun part. This chapter is dedicated to all the delicious foods that can provide protection against stroke and other modern diseases—foods such as fruits, vegetables, whole grains, meats, poultry, fish, nuts, beans, lentils, certain vegetable oils, and low-fat dairy. It also contains sections on beverages, condiments, and even sweeteners that may be included in a healthy diet.

Throughout this chapter, you will find AHA dietary recommendations for a variety of foods. The diet most similar to the AHA diet, which is aimed at lowering risks of both heart attack and stroke, is the Mediterranean diet. (See inset on page 207.) Appropriately, there is robust evidence that following the Mediterranean diet can aid in stroke prevention.

WHOLE GRAINS

As mentioned in the previous chapter, it is a good idea to opt for foods made with whole grains and avoid white flour and other foods that have been stripped of most of their nutrients by food manufacturers. The AHA diet recommends three to four servings of whole grains each day. (One serving generally consists of 1/2 cup of cooked grains, 1 slice of whole grain bread, or 1 ounce of whole grain cereal.) Eating at least three servings of whole grains has been shown to decrease the risks of age-related diseases, including heart disease (by 25 to 36 percent), stroke (by 37 percent), type 2 diabetes (by 21 to 27 percent), certain cancers, and obesity. Only 4 percent of American adults, however, consume at least three servings of whole grains daily.

Whole grains are important because every whole grain kernel consists of bran, endosperm, and germ, each of which contains different nutrients. When these kernels are milled, most of the bran and some of the germ are lost in the process, leaving white flour. Nutrients found in whole grains include B vitamins, vitamin E, iron, copper, magnesium, zinc, selenium, essential fatty acids, and fiber. Whole grains may also contain healthy phyotchemicals such as lignans, flavonoids, phenolic acids, carotenoids, and phytosteroids. Whole wheat, bulgur, wheat berries, rye, dried corn, brown rice, amaranth, faro, and quinoa are common examples of whole grains.

There are many whole grain products to choose from—breads, cereals, crackers, pasta, wraps, tacos, and so on. When purchasing a product made with whole grains, make sure the label states, "100% whole grain." If it states, "wheat flour," it is not true whole wheat. If a product boasts that it "contains whole wheat," the product may contain mostly refined wheat and could be only 1 percent whole wheat.

FRUITS AND VEGETABLES

The AHA recommends at least five servings of a variety of fruits and vegetables (one serving generally consists of 1/2 cup of most fruits and vegetables, or 1 cup of leafy greens) each day to reduce the risk of stroke and cardiovascular disease. Research suggests even better results when people consume ten servings a day. Specifically, a British study looked at two million people by consolidating ninety-five other studies. Consuming ten servings of fruits and vegetables was associated with significant reductions in risks of heart disease (by 24 percent), stroke (by 33 percent), cardiovascular disease (by 28 percent), total cancer (by 13 percent), and premature death (by 31 percent). The lead author commented that there is no way to put the vast array of beneficial compounds into a pill. He said, "Most likely it is the whole package of beneficial nutrients you obtain by eating fruits and vegetables that is crucial to health. This is why it is important to eat whole plant foods to get the benefit."

These scientists also looked at different groups of fruits and vegetables to see if any in particular stood out as being protective against strokes. They reported that apples, pears, citrus fruits, green leafy vegetables (spinach, lettuce, and chicory), and cruciferous vegetables (broccoli, cabbage, and cauliflower) may help prevent heart disease, stroke, and early death.

Fruits and vegetables contain a large number of healthy substances, including fiber, vitamins, minerals, enzymes, and different phytochemicals, which give fruits and vegetables their colors and also affect their tastes and smells. While brightly colored fruits and vegetables possess antioxidant properties, allowing them to neutralize free radicals and protect against strokes, white fruits and vegetables are also associated with a lower risk of stroke. Each different fruit and vegetable contains a unique set of nutrients, so variety may be the key to reaping their benefits as fully as possible.

Fruits

Fruits are naturally low in fat, sodium, and calories. None has cholesterol. They supply many essential nutrients that are under-consumed in the United States and other Western countries, including potassium, dietary fiber, vitamin C, vitamin A, and folic acid. Potassium is important for maintaining healthy blood pressure and normal heart rhythm. Dietary fiber helps reduce cholesterol and may lower heart disease risk. Foods that are high in fiber promote feelings of fullness without being high in calories and encourage healthy bowel movements.

Different groups of fruits contain different phytochemicals. If you choose fruits from different groups, you will be getting a variety of phytochemicals. For example, citrus fruits contain an abundance of flavonoids, while berries are rich in anthocyanins.

Whole fruit is a better choice than juice. For example, flavonoids are especially found in the white pith of citrus fruit. In fact, if you eat a whole orange, you will be getting five times more flavonoids than you would by drinking eight ounces of orange juice. Both oranges and orange juice, however, have been associated with fewer strokes.

Scientists have reported that berries contain some of the most powerful disease-fighting chemicals, with high antioxidant levels and anthocyanins, which are responsible for their blue, black, and red colors. These substances also reduce risk factors for cardiovascular disease and type 2 diabetes.

A mixture of blueberries, blackberries, raspberries, and strawberries in an attractive bowl is a sight to behold and delicious to eat. If the berries are too sour to eat, just add a little of one of the sweeteners mentioned on page 211. Watermelon is a rich a source of lycopene, a powerful antioxidant, which is thought to reduce the risk of stroke by almost 20 percent. Tomatoes are also a great source of lycopene. The higher the level of lycopene in the blood, the lower the risk of stroke. When you cook tomatoes, you reduce their vitamin C content, but you get a much bigger boost of lycopene from them. So, products such as canned tomato purée, canned cooked tomatoes, and spaghetti sauce are good sources of lycopene. When shopping for these times, however, look for low-sodium versions. If possible, make tomato sauce from scratch, since canned and bottled versions typically have added sugar, salt, and preservatives.

Apples and pears should be eaten whole (except their cores) because many of antioxidants and phytochemicals are found in their skins. Anthocyanins give red apples their color and have anti-inflammatory, anti-viral, and anti-cancer effects. The old saying, "An apple a day keeps the doctor away" may be true! In fact, one researcher suggested, "An apple a day may keep a stroke away!"

There is a wealth of different phytochemicals in kiwis, including carotenoids and flavonoids. Kiwis can protect cells from oxidative stress but may also increase HDL (good cholesterol), decrease triglycerides, and lower blood pressure.

Fruits contain so many beneficial substances that it is difficult to determine the exact mechanism that makes high fruit intake protective against stroke. It is also hard to pinpoint exactly which fruits offer the most protection. As such, it is best to choose a wide variety of fruits of different colors. Fruit is a reasonable way to enjoy sweetness while avoiding refined sugar and other unhealthy ingredients.

GLYCEMIC INDEX AND GLYCEMIC LOAD

The glycemic index (GI) is a ranking system of the carbohydrates found in different foods. It is meant to help determine how a food will affect blood glucose levels. It lists foods on a scale of 0 to 100, with higher values corresponding to higher and quicker rises in blood sugar, and with a low GI value being 55 or less. Essentially, it determines the quality of a food's carbohydrates. When trying to manage blood sugar levels, however, a food's GI value, or quality of a food's carbohydrates, may be a less helpful measurement than its glycemic load (GL) number.

The glycemic load (GL) reflects not only the glycemic index of a food but also the amount of carbohydrates contained in a designated portion of food, providing a measurement that includes both the quality and quantity of a food's carbohydrates. The GL of a food is calculated through a simple mathematical formula. The food's GI value is multiplied by the number of carbohydrates (in grams) contained in a given portion of that food and then divided by 100. Values of 20 or more are considered high, numbers of 11 through 19 fall in the medium range, and numbers of 10 or less are regarded as low. A daily GL of 80 or less is considered low, while a GL of 120 or more falls in the high range.

In general, it is best to aim for a low glycemic load. Tips for doing so include eating more vegetables and fruits, choosing foods with higher fiber contents, eating whole grains, limiting processed foods, cutting down on foods with added sugar, and eating smaller portions.

Vegetables

Like fruits, most vegetables are naturally low in fat and calories and contain no cholesterol. Vegetables also provide a variety of essential nutrients, including potassium, dietary fiber, folate, vitamin A in the form of beta-carotene, vitamin C, vitamin K, and dietary fiber. Lastly, vegetables are a rich source of phytochemicals. Just think of the yellow in yellow squash, the orange in pumpkin and sweet potatoes, the green that masks the color of many orange-yellow carotenoids present in green leafy vegetables, the red in beets, or the purple in purple cabbage. As you know, when produce is vividly colored, it's full of health-promoting phytochemicals—although white vegetables are important, too, and contain certain other phytochemicals.

When it comes to leafy greens, the darker the green in leafy vegetables, the richer the nutrients. Leafy greens can be steamed, used to make salads, or added to whole grain bowls. When making salads or coleslaw, mix in purple cabbage along with green cabbage, or use only red cabbage. Purple cabbage is ten times as rich in vitamin A as green cabbage, and its high potassium content helps lower blood pressure. Purple cabbage also brightens up a plate. When food looks attractive, it is eaten more enthusiastically.

They can also be used to make smoothies. Just throw some kale or spinach in a blender along with milk and purée. You can substitute yogurt for milk (it's better for you) and add fruit for sweetness (e.g., berries). You can add a spoonful of almond butter for protein. You won't even realize you're drinking your fruits and vegetables for breakfast.

When eating potatoes, remember that sweet potatoes have a lower glycemic index than white potatoes. And make sure you eat their skins, too. The skin of a potato contains even more nutrients than its interior and about half of its total fiber content. When making mashed potatoes, don't peel the potatoes. In addition, avoid French fries, hash browns, loaded potato skins, and greasy potatoes.

The onion family of vegetables (onions, garlic, leeks, shallots, scallions, and chives) has sulfur compounds that can act as natural blood thinners, which can help prevent blood clots. When eaten raw, these vegetables have also displayed the ability to lower blood pressure.

When choosing vegetables to eat, it is better to opt for vegetables with low glycemic loads. A rule of thumb to determine the glycemic loads of vegetables is to determine whether they grow above or below ground. Vegetables that grow below ground, such as root vegetables (potatoes, carrots, turnips, parsnip, etc.) have higher glycemic loads than those that grow above ground (broccoli, broccolini, leafy greens, etc.). People who are overweight, obese, prediabetic, or diabetic, should limit their consumption of root vegetables and eat more above-ground vegetables.

Just like we don't know everything about fruits, there is still much to be learned about vegetables and all their benefits. Nevertheless, we do know that a diet high in vegetables helps reduce the risks of stroke and other serious disorders. Foods such as dark leafy greens, broccoli, Brussels sprouts, sweet potatoes, onions, garlic, carrots, beets, and squash are a crucial part of any anti-stroke diet.

WHAT IS SOFRITO?

Sofrito is a widely used tomato sauce for meat, fish, pasta, and vegetables. It's used in cooking by many different cultures and in many different countries with diverse added spices. It is often served over rice and beans and in soups, chili, or stews. The Mediterranean diet—widely known for its ability to lower stroke risk—recommends that you use 1/2 cup several times a week.

To make sofrito, place 4 diced tomatoes, 1/2 large chopped onion, 2 pressed garlic cloves, 1/2 tablespoon dried basil, and 2 tablespoons extra virgin olive oil in a saucepan and bring them to a simmer. Cover and simmer for as many hours as desired. Add a little water if the sauce becomes too thick. Experiment with other vegetables and spices such as bell peppers, oregano, and cilantro.

If a stroke patient is unable to make sofrito himself, a relative or friend could prepare a batch for him to keep in his refrigerator. Sofrito can also be purchased online. It is an enjoyable way to reduce stroke risk.

DAIRY PRODUCTS AND ALTERNATIVES

The American Heart Association recommends consuming two to three servings of low-fat dairy products, which include milk, cheese, and yogurt, every day. One serving generally consists of 1 cup of milk or yogurt, or 1.5 ounces of cheese. Regular consumption of dairy foods lowers the risk of obesity, prediabetes, type 2 diabetes, high blood pressure, and heart disease. Two reviews of a number of studies showed that dairy products were protective against stroke. The beneficial effects of dairy products are not fully understood but may be due to several factors, including their short- and medium-chain fatty acids, probiotics, and vitamins and minerals (e.g., calcium, vitamin A, vitamin B_2, vitamin B_3, vitamin B_{12}, vitamin D, potassium, and phosphorus), and protein.

Although we have assumed for decades that dairy fat is unhealthy, and despite the fact that the AHA recommends consuming low-fat dairy, there is a growing body of scientific evidence that suggests that dairy fat does not increase the risk of cardiovascular disease. Recent studies have found that whole-fat dairy does not cause weight gain; dairy consumption improves body composition by increasing lean body mass and reducing body fat; yogurt consumption reduces weight gain; fermented dairy, including cheese, lowers cardiovascular risk; and yogurt, cheese, and even dairy fat protect against type 2 diabetes.

Dairy products are excellent sources of important nutrients. One cup of skim milk has 8 grams of protein, containing all the essential amino acids. If you consume a 2,000-calorie diet each day, one cup of skim milk will provide 50 percent of your daily calcium needs, 20 percent of recommended vitamin B_2, 16 percent of recommended vitamin B_{12}, 25 percent of recommended phosphorous, and 12 percent of recommended potassium, and only 86 calories. One glass of whole milk contains 146 calories due to its 5 grams of saturated fat. Milk is also fortified with vitamin D, which is critical for bone health.

Those who avoid dairy milk and other dairy products, whether due to allergy, lactose intolerance, or personal preference, should try to get similar nutrition from alternatives to dairy milk, which include almond milk, coconut milk, rice milk, soy milk, hemp milk, and oat milk. This is particularly true in the case of calcium, especially if osteoporosis or osteopenia is present. Milk substitutes may not have the same amounts of nutrients as dairy milk, however, so whether they reduce stroke risk is questionable. They also typically have higher sugar contents than milk, so make sure to read labels.

Yogurt is another dairy product that offers many nutrients. One cup of plain low-fat yogurt has about 154 calories, 2.5 grams of saturated fat, and almost 13 grams of protein. One cup provides about 45 percent of daily calcium needs, 10 percent of recommended magnesium, 35 percent of recommended phosphorous, 16 percent of recommended potassium, 15 percent of recommended zinc, and 12 percent of recommended selenium. Yogurt contains vitamin D only if it has been fortified, which should be marked on its label. Be sure to read the label of any yogurt you buy to make sure it does not have added sugars or artificial sweeteners. In the United States, yogurt is typically eaten sweet (with added sugar or fruit), but other cultures enjoy even healthier savory yogurt dishes, such as Greek yogurt mixed with diced cucumbers, salt, pepper, and dried mint.

Some dairy products are high in saturated fat (e.g., sour cream, cream cheese, heavy cream, buttermilk , etc.) and high in calories, and should be eaten rarely, and even then in modest amounts if you are overweight or obese. And what about butter? Butter is made from animal fat, so it contains saturated fat. If you ask most doctors, they will tell you to use margarine and avoid butter. But the truth is there is no good evidence that using butter increases the risk of heart attack or stroke. If you like olive oil, definitely use it instead of butter on bread or for flavoring. Another possibility is to use butter that is combined with olive oil or canola oil, which lowers the total saturated fats but retains some of the butter taste. In addition, whipped butter has less saturated fat and calories per tablespoon.

Margarine, on the other hand, contains vegetable oil, so it should be healthier. Unfortunately, not all margarines are created equal. Avoid any product that lists partially hydrogenated oil in its ingredient list, as this term means it contains trans fat, even though the Nutrition Facts label may list the trans fat content as zero. Those patients with high cholesterol should ask their doctors if they should use a spread fortified with plant sterols and stanols. These substances, also found naturally in fruits, vegetables, vegetable oils, legumes, and nuts, block absorption of cholesterol in the large intestine, lowering cholesterol in the blood. Butter or margarine consumption should not exceed 1 tablespoon a day, due to the number of calories these products contain.

LEAN MEAT, POULTRY, AND EGGS

In a balanced diet, protein is a key requirement. Protein requirements are based on weight: Men need about 56 grams of protein per day, while women need about 46 grams per day. When you eat foods containing protein, your digestive juices break it down into smaller units called amino acids. In fact, amino acids are referred to as the "building blocks" of protein. There are nine essential amino acids that your body cannot make, so they must be attained from dietary sources. All nine are found in meat, poultry, eggs, and fish. Although lean meat, poultry, and eggs are sources of protein, necessary proteins can be found in non-animal sources. Non-animal sources of all nine amino acids include quinoa, which is a grain, and soybean, which is a legume. While nuts, leafy green vegetables, and most grains and legumes do not contain all nine essential amino acids, if you combine these foods in a meal, you should be able to get all of them to make a complete protein—and without any saturated fat or cholesterol. In other words, you don't need to get all your protein from animal sources.

Although red meat is an important source of protein, essential amino acids, vitamins, and minerals, it also contains more cholesterol and saturated fat than chicken, fish, or vegetables. A high consumption of red meat has been associated with a greater risk of stroke, cardiovascular death, and certain types of cancer. Consumption of processed meat (ham, sausage, bacon, luncheon meat, and hot dogs) leads to an even greater risk of major age-related diseases, including stroke. The American Heart Association recommends limiting red meats (beef, pork, and lamb) as they have more saturated fat than chicken, fish, or vegetable protein. The unsaturated fat in fish is actually good for you. Omega-3-fatty acids, found in fish and some plants, are part of a heart-and-brain-healthy diet. Stroke patients and at-risk individuals are advised to reduce the amount of steak, hamburger, and processed meat in their diets, replacing these foods with healthier protein-rich options such as poultry without the skin, turkey, tofu, beans, or fish. (See Table 12.1. Protein-Rich Foods on page 206.) This change can greatly reduce stroke risk.

Eggs are another good source of protein and many other nutrients. The yolk is a rich source of phytochemicals. Yes, eggs are one of the richest dietary sources of cholesterol, but they also contain nutrients that may lower the risk of heart disease and stroke. In addition, dietary cholesterol is only weakly related to blood cholesterol. Most of the cholesterol in your blood is actually made by your body.

So, should you consume eggs or not? The cardiovascular studies of eating eggs have shown conflicting results, leaving patients and even doctors puzzled. Some studies suggest that eating an egg every day does not cause more strokes or heart attacks. These same studies, however, also suggest that eating eggs every day may be associated with an elevated risk of heart failure in men and type 2 diabetes in the general population. Conversely, a study of 500,000 adults reported that eating one egg per day led to a lower risk of heart disease and stroke, but the adults were Chinese and did not consume a Western diet. Whether or not the results apply to Westerners is unknown.

One egg or two eggs whites may be considered one serving as part of a healthy diet for people who like eggs. If possible, buy eggs that were produced by hens fed an omega-3 enriched diet, as these provide five times as much omega-3s as conventional eggs. Keep in mind that prolonged heat and exposure to oxygen damage the cholesterol, starting a process that can lead to plaque formation in the blood vessels. Therefore, prepare eggs by poaching or soft-boiling rather than frying or scrambling. Hard-boiled eggs are fine, too, because the shell protects the egg from oxygen. And don't eat eggs with unhealthy foods such as bacon or sausage, which will increase the risk of stroke.

TABLE 12.1. PROTEIN-RICH FOODS

Food	Serving Size	Protein
Round steak	3 ounces	23 g
Tuna, salmon, trout	3 ounces	21g
Turkey, chicken	3 ounces	19 g
Greek yogurt	6 ounces	17 g
Cottage cheese	1/2 cup	17 g
Lentils	1/2 cup	12 g
Tofu	4 ounces	10 g
Cooked beans	1/2 cup	8 g
Milk	1 cup	8 g
Quinoa	1 cup	8 g
Cooked whole wheat pasta	1 cup	7 g
Nuts	1/4 cup	7 g
Eggs	1 egg	6 g

MEDITERRANEAN DIET REDUCES RISK OF STROKE

The traditional Mediterranean diet is characterized by high intakes of vegetables, legumes, fruits, nuts, cereals (mostly unrefined), and olive oil; moderate intake of fish; low-to-moderate intake of dairy products (mostly in the form of cheese or yogurt); low intakes of saturated fat, meat, and poultry; and moderate intake of alcohol (primarily in the form of wine during meals).

In light of the fact that several large studies had shown that people who follow a Mediterranean diet have fewer strokes and heart attacks than those who do not, a landmark study in Spain known as the PRED-IMED study decided to compare followers of two different versions of the Mediterranean diet with followers of a low-fat diet. In this study, 7,447 participants with high cardiovascular risk were recruited, randomly assigned to one of the three diets, and monitored for occurrence of stroke, heart attack, and death. The first diet was a Mediterranean diet supplemented with extra virgin olive oil; the second diet was a Mediterranean diet supplemented with mixed nuts; the third was a low fat diet.

After approximately five years, those who had consumed either version of the Mediterranean diet had a lower risk of a combined measure of heart attack, stroke, and death from cardiovascular causes compared with those who had consumed the low-fat diet. The study also found that the overall benefit was driven mainly by the reduction in stroke risk, which suggests that following this type of diet is a powerful way to prevent strokes. This study is the best evidence to date of an ideal anti-stroke diet.

SEAFOOD

Seafood is a key component of the Mediterranean diet. The AHA recommends two to three servings of seafood each week. (One serving consists of 3 ounces of fish.) Seafood is a great source of protein and healthy fat. Avoid frying fish. Instead, it can be sautéed in a little olive oil, baked, or broiled. Good seafood options include omega-3-rich fish such as albacore tuna, salmon, sardines, herring, and other fatty fish. The fat in these fish are healthy. Cod, catfish, clams, scallops, and shrimp are also healthy choices, even if they are not great sources of omega-3s.

LEGUMES, NUTS, AND SEEDS

The American Heart Association recommends four to five servings of legumes, nuts, or seeds each week as part of a healthy diet. (One serving consists of 1/2 cup of cooked beans or peas, or 2 tablespoons of nuts or seeds.)

Legumes, which include beans, green beans, peas, and lentils, are truly super foods. They are low in price but high in vitamins, minerals, protein, essential fatty acids, fiber, and a variety of phytochemicals. Legumes could actually be listed in both the vegetable and protein groups of foods. Surprisingly, however, there does not seem to be evidence that eating beans lowers stroke risk. Nevertheless, legumes have been shown to decrease insulin levels, improve metabolic syndrome and prediabetes, lower body weight, lower cholesterol, and reduce high blood pressure—all risk factors for stroke. So, eating beans dishes several times a week is a good idea.

Beans can be used in salads, soups, side dishes, and entrées. Great Northern beans, kidney beans, navy beans, and soybeans all contain significant amounts of omega-3 fatty acids. Beans that you cook yourself are the healthiest choice because you can control the amount of salt being used, but if you prefer the convenience of canned beans, choose low-sodium brands or place the beans in a sieve and rinse them thoroughly under cold running water to wash away as much of the sodium as possible before using them.

Beans contain certain sugars that the body does not completely break down, leading to excessive gas production and bloating. Thankfully, soaking or sprouting the beans before cooking them can prevent this problem.

Nuts and seeds are little packets chock full of many nutrients. Nuts and seeds are high in protein, vitamin E, beta-carotene, B vitamins, calcium, copper, magnesium, phosphorus, selenium, essential fatty acids, and fiber. Although there have been mixed results in regard to their decreasing the risk of stroke, nuts have been found to lower cholesterol and triglycerides, decrease fasting blood sugar, decrease inflammation, and reduce the risk of heart disease. As they combat these health conditions related to stroke, nuts—such as almonds, walnuts, hazelnuts, pecans, pine nuts, and pistachios—and seeds—such as sesame seeds, chia seeds, flaxseeds, hemp seeds, and pumpkin seeds—are a wise dietary choice.

Nuts should be purchased in their raw, unsalted form and stored in a cool, dry place. Roasted nuts should be avoided, as high heat destroys some of their nutrients. Remember that 80 percent of a nut is made up of fat, and even though most of this fat is beneficial, it still means nuts are high in calories—about 260 calories in 1.5 ounces—so don't overindulge.

Advice for Caregivers
HELPING A STROKE SURVIVOR WITH HIS MENU

Once your loved one is able to choose foods and beverages to eat, point him in the direction of the healthy foods on his menu in the hospital and rehabilitation unit. Encourage him to opt for lots of fruits and vegetables, dark green salads, whole grain breads and cereals, poultry, and fish. Keep red meats to a minimum. If you will be eating meals with him, be sure to choose similar foods. Don't bring fast food, sugary beverages, or candy for him or yourself.

VEGETABLE OILS AND DRESSINGS

As discussed in Chapter 10, omega-3 fatty acids and omega-6 fatty acids are protective against a variety of cardiovascular diseases. These essential fatty acids can be found in vegetable oil, which can also provide decent amounts of vitamin E, vitamin K, and phytochemicals.

The AHA diet recommends two to three servings of vegetable oil a day. (One serving consists of 1 tablespoon of vegetable oil.) It suggests using extra virgin olive oil, based on the results of the PREDIMED study (see inset on page 207) and various other studies of the Mediterranean diet. While olive oil does not contain a large amount of omega-3 or omega-6 fatty acids, it does contain a high level of oleic acid, an omega-9 fatty acid that has been associated with inflammation reduction. Olive oil also contains other chemicals that act as strong antioxidants. It can lower blood pressure, help control blood sugar and insulin sensitivity, lower LDL cholesterol, and boost HDL cholesterol. Other healthy options include canola or walnut oil, as both are high in omega-3 fatty acids.

The omega-3 and omega-6 fatty acids in vegetable oil are fragile and can be damaged by high temperatures, so sautéing foods at low temperatures is recommended when using it to cook. Olive oil can also be used in salad dressings or to flavor cooked vegetables, fish, or chicken.

CONDIMENTS

Condiments can add color and flavor to many foods. Some condiments are good for you because they are rich in phytochemicals or other healthy ingredients, while others are unhealthy because of too much added salt, sugar, corn syrup, or artificial colors and flavors. (See Table 12.2. Choosing Condiments below.) The Nutrition Facts label on any condiment will show you how much salt and sugar are present in a serving, and the Ingredients list will note any sweeteners or artificial colors and flavors. If you want your condiments to be as healthy as possible, make them at home. You can find simple recipes online.

TABLE 12.2. CHOOSING CONDIMENTS

Condiments	Healthy Ingredients	Recommendation
Ketchup	Tomatoes, vinegar, spices	Avoid brands high in salt, sugar, or high-fructose corn syrup
Relish	Vegetables, vinegar	Avoid brands high in salt, corn syrup, or food dye
Mustard	Mustard seed	Avoid brands high in salt or food dye
Mayonnaise	Oil (choose olive oil mayo), eggs, vinegar	Remember mayonnaise is very high in calories
Salsa	Vegetables, occasionally fruit, herbs, spices	Avoid brands high in salt

Herbs and spices can also be considered condiments. When purchasing herbs or spices, avoid ones with added salt.

SWEETENERS

Sugar—in all its many forms—is highly damaging to your health. Artificial sweeteners, although non-caloric, can have their own adverse effects on the body. All sweeteners are addictive and stimulate the brain to want even more sweetness and to eat even more food than the body actually requires. In an ideal world, perhaps no one would consume added sweeteners, but we don't live in an ideal, sugar-free world. Thankfully, there are sweeteners you can try that are safer than others. Even when using these sweeteners, however, it is advisable to use the smallest amount possible. Your brain, heart, and body will thank you for doing so.

Stevia is a natural sweetener that contains zero calories. Some people object to its slightly bitter or licorice taste, although others love it. In one study, diabetics who used stevia for sixty days were found to have lower fasting blood sugar than subjects that did not use stevia.

Monk fruit, like stevia, is many times sweeter than cane sugar, so only a small amount should be used. And like stevia, it also has zero calories and will not affect blood glucose levels.

Xylitol is a sugar substitute but it is not completely calorie-free. It can be digested and absorbed to some extent. Like its cousin sorbitol, xylitol may cause digestive problems such as diarrhea, gas, or bloating. The effect is often dose-related, so xylitol use should be decreased if gastrointestinal problems arise. Xylitol is poisonous to dogs, possibly leading to low blood sugar, liver failure, or even death, so it should be kept away from these four-legged friends. It is important to note that dogs are especially attracted to sugar-free gum. Xylitol powder may be found in most health food stores, some groceries, and online.

Unprocessed honey is another sweetener that may be used safely in small amounts. We're not talking about ordinary supermarket honey, which has been heated and filtered, removing most of the nutrients. We're referring to locally grown organic raw honey, which may be found in health food stores, farmers' markets, and online. Dark-colored honey is preferred, as it contains more antioxidants than light-colored honey.

In general, studies have shown that raw honey is preferable to refined sugar as a sweetener. Natural honey has been used as a healing substance since ancient times and contains more than 180 biologically active substances. According to scientists, natural honey has antibacterial, antifungal, antivirus, anti-inflammatory, antihypertensive, antioxidant, and antitumor properties, and is protective of the heart and liver. It may also lower blood sugar.

Natural honey may benefit patients with cardiovascular disease, as it seems to have the ability to reduce body weight mildly; decrease triglycerides, total cholesterol, and LDL cholesterol; and increase HDL cholesterol.

It is very important to note that children younger than one year of age should never be given honey, as an infant's underdeveloped immune system cannot handle the spores it may contain.

BEVERAGES

Although drinking beverages containing sugar, high-fructose corn syrup, or artificial sweeteners may increase stroke risk, some beverages can actually decrease this risk, including coffee, tea, cocoa, and even alcohol in moderation. Coffee, tea, and cocoa are important sources of polyphenols, which seem to reduce the risk of stroke because they lower blood pressure and cholesterol while providing antioxidant and anti-inflammatory effects. They also seem to protect the lining of blood vessels.

In the past, coffee was considered a risk factor for cardiovascular disease. Recent studies, however, suggest that moderate coffee consumption, which translates to three to four cups a day, may reduce stroke risk. Coffee contains hundreds of biologically active chemicals, including polyphenols and caffeine. While caffeine causes an immediate rise in systolic and diastolic blood pressure, over time this effect decreases. Studies show that moderate coffee consumption may reduce both ischemic and hemorrhagic stroke risks.

Green tea and black tea are the most commonly consumed beverages in the world. Tea is produced from the leaves of the plant *Camellia sinensis* and is classified by the degree of fermentation: black tea (fermented); oolong tea (partially fermented); and green tea (unfermented). In studies, men and women who consumed four or more cups of black or green tea a day had approximately 20 percent lower risk of stroke than those who did not drink tea. All types of tea are rich in flavonoids, which have both strong antioxidant and anti-inflammatory effects. Tea and tea-derived flavonoids may have beneficial effects on the lining of blood vessels. They may also lower blood pressure, cholesterol, and blood glucose. In addition, tea has a calming effect, so a cup of hot tea or a tall glass of refreshing iced tea can be helpful to an individual suffering from anxiety.

Products made from cacao or cocoa, such as chocolate, are also rich sources of flavonoids. Numerous studies have reported links between chocolate or cocoa consumption and reduced fasting insulin levels and improved linings of blood vessels, while demonstrating no effects on cholesterol or triglycerides. Stroke risk seems to decrease in association with chocolate consumption. So, a cup of hot cocoa may be a good idea for those at risk of or recovering from a stroke, as long as it has been made without sugar (try a little xylitol or unprocessed honey instead).

The association between alcohol consumption and stroke risk is tricky. Moderate amounts of alcohol (one or fewer drinks per day for women, and two or fewer drinks per day for men) may actually be protective against stroke—and this benefit is associated with any type of alcohol, not just wine, which is well known as a key component of the healthy Mediterranean diet. If a person drinks more than moderately, however, then alcohol consumption no longer has a protective effect and instead increases the risk of stroke substantially. In fact, heavy alcohol use is one of the biggest risk factors for a hemorrhagic (or bleeding) stroke. For this reason, we generally don't recommend that those who do not normally drink suddenly begin drinking regularly. In addition, those with a history of alcoholism or binge drinking should avoid drinking altogether. Those who would like to have a drink with dinner and have never had a hemorrhagic stroke, of course, are fine to do so.

CONCLUSION

It's exciting to know that simply by changing your diet, you can greatly reduce your stroke risk—and your risk of all the other age-related diseases. Nevertheless, change is not easy. Most people would find replacing their current eating habits with an anti-stroke diet to be a very intimidating task. Fortunately, the next chapter provides sample meal plans that will make the transition to a healthier lifestyle a little easier. It even includes ideas for wholesome snacks and guidance on how to make wise dietary choices outside the home.

13

*F*ollowing the Anti-Stroke Diet

Over the last three chapters, you learned about the nutritional components that make foods healthy, which foods are rich in these heart-healthy and brain-healthy nutrients, and which foods to limit or avoid to stroke risk. Now it's time to put all this information into action.

This chapter reviews the basics of the anti-stroke diet and offers a week's worth of daily menus that feature wholesome meals and snacks built around these basic ideas. It also explains how to make snacks that are nutritionally worthwhile but also satisfying, providing examples of snacks that are packed with vitamins, minerals, and other healthy substances yet free of anti-nutrients that can sabotage their health benefits. Finally, it offers tips on dining out so that you can enjoy nourishing, health-promoting meals when eating outside the home. You will find that eating well is a big part of preventing strokes.

THE BASICS

Following the anti-stroke diet isn't complicated, but it does mean organizing meals and snacks so that all the fruits, vegetables, lean proteins, whole grains, and other foods required for good health are included over the course of a day. It also means avoiding processed foods that are high in salt or sugar and nutritionally empty. While this task may seem challenging, the results will be worth the effort, as eating the right diet can help sharply reduce stroke risk.

In an effective anti-stroke diet, which is generally based on the Mediterranean diet, dietary goals include:

- 3 servings of fresh fruit a day

- 2 or more servings of vegetables a day

- 3 or more servings of fish (especially fatty fish) or seafood a week

- 3 or more servings of legumes a week

- 2 servings of sofrito a week

- choosing white meat instead of red meat

- 4 tablespoons of olive oil a day

- 3 or more servings of tree nuts a week

The American Heart Association diet, from which the anti-stroke diet draws many of its guidelines, also includes whole grains and low-fat dairy products while limiting salt intake. An effective anti-stroke diet also limits soda and other sugary drinks (less than one serving a day); baked goods, sweets, and pastries (fewer than three servings a week); fatty spreads (less than one serving a day); and red or processed meat (less than one serving a day).

Now that you know which foods to choose in your effort to prevent a stroke, you are ready to plan meals. Visualize a dinner-sized plate for each meal. Half the plate should be filled with fruits and vegetables. One quarter should contain protein—fish, chicken, or legumes—and the final fourth should contain whole grains. Add a large salad of dark green leafy greens and one or two tablespoons of a tasty salad dressing made with extra virgin olive oil. Although olive oil doesn't contain nearly as much omega-3 content as canola or walnut oil, it can still lower the risks of heart disease, high blood pressure, and stroke. A serving of milk, yogurt, or cheese may be included twice a day. For those who would like an occasional drink, women can enjoy a glass of wine each day, and men can have two glasses. The website ChooseMyPlate (www.choosemyplate.gov), which is run by the US Department of Agriculture, offers helpful tips and visuals on eating healthy.

Another way to proceed is to aim to eat five servings of fruit and vegetables daily, counting them off in your head—or on paper—as you eat them. Vegetables can even be eaten at breakfast time. A smoothie made with yogurt, banana, strawberries, and kale will provide a milk product, fruits, and a vegetable. It doesn't really matter which meal or snack is eaten, but rather that these standards are followed each day. In relation to whole grains, eating oatmeal at breakfast has been shown to lower stroke risk.

Of course, different people have different dietary needs, and certain health conditions may make it necessary to limit consumption of certain foods. These are only a few of the reasons to consult with a doctor or dietitian before beginning any diet, including the one outlined in this book.

THE MENUS

The menus that begin on page 218 create a comprehensive guide on how to follow the anti-stroke diet for a full week. Each day's plan includes three meals and three snacks. Serving sizes are also included to ensure healthy amounts of grains, proteins, nuts, dairy products, and oils are consumed. When it comes to fruits and vegetables, try to get at least five servings every day, but more fruits and vegetables are allowed as long as other types of healthful food are included in your meal plan. Fruits and vegetables are important, but legumes, protein, grains, and nuts should not be forgotten.

Remember that a serving of vegetables doesn't only mean a bowl of salad or a side dish of cooked veggies. A cup of vegetable soup, a glass of low-sodium tomato juice, or a ladle of tomato sauce or sofrito (see page 202) on pasta also counts as a serving. Another option is to incorporate several servings of both vegetables and fruits in a creamy breakfast (or lunch) smoothie.

As long as the guidelines provided on page 216 are followed, any food on a daily menu may be replaced by a different food in the same category (protein, vegetables, dairy, etc.). To get the most nutrition out of meals, the most colorful fruits and vegetables should be included, as these are the ones that are packed with extra healthy nutrients. (If you're not sure which foods offer the greatest nutritional benefits, turn back to Chapter 12 on page 196.)

Be aware that the diet outlined in this chapter provides about 2,000 calories each day, but it can be modified to provide extra calories as needed. Preferably, calories should be added in the forms of lean protein, like white meat chicken and fish, and foods rich in healthy fats, like nuts and olive oil. As necessary, more generous portions of the most wholesome forms of carbohydrates, such as brown rice, quinoa, and whole grain bread, may be provided. Low-fat yogurt and cheese may be swapped out for their full-fat counterparts if more calories are required.

Another good way to add calories to a menu plan is to supplement regular meals with smoothies that combine Greek yogurt with fruit and veggies. This will also increase protein intake. Stroke patients should always discuss their caloric needs and other nutritional requirements with their healthcare providers.

SAMPLE MENUS

DAY 1

BREAKFAST

1 poached egg

1 slice whole grain toast (spread with 1 or 2 teaspoons whipped butter if desired)

1 orange, cut into segments

1 cup cocoa (milk, cocoa powder, allowed sweetener)

1 cup coffee or tea

MORNING SNACK

½ cup strawberries

1½ ounces walnuts

LUNCH

Turkey sandwich (3 ounces roast turkey on 2 slices whole grain bread with lettuce, 2 teaspoons mustard, and 1 tablespoon olive oil mayonnaise)

1 cup lentil soup

1 cup red grapes

½ cup carrot sticks

½ cup cherry tomatoes

1 cup coffee or tea

AFTERNOON SNACK

1 cup plain low-fat Greek yogurt

½ cup blueberries

DINNER

3 ounces grilled salmon

1 baked sweet potato

½ cup steamed broccoli

Salad made with 1 cup dark leafy greens, tossed with 1 tablespoon olive oil and balsamic vinegar or lemon juice

1 wedge cantaloupe

1 cup coffee or tea

EVENING SNACK

1 cup low-sodium tomato juice

DAY 2

BREAKFAST

Smoothie made with 1 cup plain low-fat Greek yogurt, 1 cup baby kale, 1 peach, ½ banana, and 2 teaspoons ground flaxseeds

½ cup oatmeal with cinnamon and approved sweetener

1 cup coffee or tea

MORNING SNACK

½ cup blueberries

LUNCH

Salad made with 2 cups romaine lettuce, 3 ounces water-packed Albacore tuna or canned salmon, 1 sliced tomato, ½ cup chickpeas, and 1 sliced hard-boiled egg, tossed with 1½ tablespoons balsamic vinegar or lemon juice and extra virgin olive oil

½ cup strawberries mixed with ½ cup orange segments

AFTERNOON SNACK

1 apple

DINNER

1 cup cooked spaghetti squash topped with 1 cup tomato sauce or sofrito made with ground turkey

1 slice whole grain bread

1 cup melon balls

EVENING SNACK

1 cup cocoa (milk, cocoa powder, allowed sweetener)

½ cup fresh raspberries

DAY 3

BREAKFAST

1 cup whole grain ready-to-eat cereal with 1 cup low-fat milk

1 poached egg

½ cup blueberries

½ cup orange segments

1 cup coffee or tea

MORNING SNACK

5 whole grain crackers

1 ½ ounces cheese

1 cup low-sodium tomato juice

LUNCH

Turkey wrap (whole wheat tortilla, 3 ounces roasted turkey, sliced apple, shredded carrots, and 1 tablespoon olive oil mayonnaise)

1 cup bean soup

1 tangerine

1 cup coffee or tea

AFTERNOON SNACK

½ cup cherry tomatoes

½ cup broccoli florets

¼ cup salsa for dipping

DINNER

3 ounces stewed, baked, or grilled chicken

½ baked acorn squash with 1 teaspoon olive oil or butter and a sprinkling of cinnamon or nutmeg

1 cup green beans with caramelized onions

EVENING SNACK

1 peach

1 to 2 one-inch squares sugar-free dark chocolate

DAY 4

BREAKFAST

½ cup oatmeal with cinnamon and a sprinkling of raisins

1 cup cocoa (milk, cocoa powder, allowed sweetener)

1 peach, sliced

1 cup coffee or tea

MORNING SNACK

5 whole grain crackers

1 tablespoon peanut or almond butter

½ cup cherry tomatoes

LUNCH

1 cup vegetable soup

3 ounces chopped cooked chicken breast mixed with 1 tablespoon olive oil mayonnaise, herbs, and spices

½ cup carrot sticks

1 banana

1 cup coffee or tea

SNACK

1 hard-boiled egg

1 cup red grapes

1 cup low-sodium tomato juice

DINNER

3 ounces grilled or baked salmon

½ cup green peas

½ cup brown rice

½ cup cooked carrots

Salad made with 1 cup raw kale, tossed with 1 tablespoon walnut oil and balsamic vinegar

1 cup mixed fresh fruit

EVENING SNACK

1 apple

1.5 ounces cheddar cheese

DAY 5

BREAKFAST

1 cup low-sodium tomato juice

1 egg, poached, soft-boiled, or hard-boiled

1 slice whole grain toast (spread with 2 teaspoons whipped butter if desired)

1 cup melon balls, orange segments, and blueberries

1 cup coffee or tea

MORNING SNACK

2 stalks celery spread with 2 tablespoons cashew butter

1 apple

LUNCH

1 cup vegetable soup

1 whole grain pita bread filled with sliced tomato, sliced cucumber, and 2 tablespoons hummus

1 cup red grapes

1 cup low-fat milk

AFTERNOON SNACK

5 whole grain crackers

1 stick string cheese

1 cup low-sodium tomato juice

DINNER

1 cup turkey chili (sofrito base) with beans

Salad made with 1 cup spinach and 1 cup shredded carrots and purple cabbage, tossed with 1 tablespoon olive oil and balsamic vinegar

1 slice watermelon

EVENING SNACK

1 cup mixed berries

1 to 2 one-inch square sugar-free dark chocolate

DAY 6

BREAKFAST

Smoothie made with 1 cup plain low-fat Greek yogurt, 1 cup baby kale, ½ banana, ½ cup fresh pineapple, ½ cup sliced strawberries, and 2 teaspoons ground flaxseeds

1 tangerine

1 cup coffee or tea

MORNING SNACK

1.5 ounces walnuts

1 cup red grapes

LUNCH

Egg salad sandwich (2 slices whole grain bread spread with 1 chopped egg, 2 teaspoons olive oil mayonnaise, and 1 teaspoon mustard, topped with romaine lettuce)

½ cup bean salad

½ cup cherries

1 cup low-fat milk

AFTERNOON SNACK

1 cup carrot sticks, celery sticks, and broccoli florets

¼ cup low-fat vegetable dip

DINNER

3 ounces grilled chicken

½ cup quinoa

Salad made with 2 cups dark leafy greens, tossed with 1½ tablespoons olive oil and balsamic vinegar

1 cup mixed berries

1 cup coffee or tea

EVENING SNACK

1 cup tomato juice

1 to 2 one-inch square sugar-free dark chocolate

DAY 7

BREAKFAST

½ cup oatmeal with ½ cup blueberries

1 cup cocoa (milk, cocoa powder, allowed sweetener)

1 cup cubed mango

1 cup coffee or tea

MORNING SNACK

1.5 ounces cheese

5 whole grain crackers

1 cup low-sodium tomato juice

LUNCH

Salad made with 2 cups romaine lettuce, 3 ounces sliced grilled chicken, ½ cup chickpeas, ½ cup halved cherry tomatoes, and ¼ cup red onion rings, tossed with 1½ tablespoons balsamic vinegar and 1 tablespoon olive oil

1 apple

AFTERNOON SNACK

1 cup cubed pineapple sprinkled with cinnamon

1 hard-boiled egg

DINNER

Veggie burger on whole wheat bun with salsa or lettuce and sliced tomato

Corn on the cob

½ cup Brussels sprouts, roasted with olive oil and garlic

1 slice watermelon

EVENING SNACK

1 cup sliced strawberries

1 cup plain low-fat Greek yogurt

Advice for Caregivers
LEFTOVERS AND EXTRA HELP

You can help your loved one create his own menus that are similar to the ones found in this chapter, but which include his preferred foods. Help him cook enough food that he will have leftovers but not so much that the food will go bad. For example, stew some chicken and then use it to make a dinner, sandwiches, or a chicken salad. The same can be done with a turkey tenderloin breast. Or bake or broil a piece of salmon to eat as a meal, using leftovers for salads or sandwiches. Hard-boil several eggs to be used for sandwiches, salads, or snacks.

When friends ask, "What can we do to help out?" find ways they can help—don't deny them the pleasure. And admit to yourself that you and your loved one could use some extra help. It could be washing a load of clothes, taking your loved one to an appointment, or simply taking him out for the day so you can rest and relax—even nap. You could ask them to bring food—low-sodium chili, a large unsweetened fruit salad, homemade low-salt broth-based soup such as bean or vegetable soup, or a favorite casserole made with the anti-stroke diet in mind. Often people want to be helpful but they don't know what is needed. Let them know.

SMART SNACK IDEAS

If you've read the menus that start on page 218, you've seen that they include three snacks in each day's meal plan. You may have been surprised, because snacking is not usually seen as a beneficial habit—especially since much of the snacking in our country involves greasy salted chips, cookies, ice cream, candy, and the like. Most common snacks are not only nutritionally empty but also provide too much saturated fat, refined sugar, or salt. Often they contain a whole day's worth of sodium. Even the best diet can be damaged in a matter of minutes by unwise snacking!

The good news is that snacking doesn't have to be unhealthy. Between-meals snacks can actually help satisfy the body's need for fruits, vegetables, and other valuable foods while also satisfying hunger. The following list includes snack ideas from the menus presented earlier and some new ideas. While all these mini-meals are packed with nutrients, when choosing snacks, it's important to keep in mind the guidelines presented on page 216. It's always a good idea to use snacks to provide needed servings of fruits and vegetables. Savory snacks on the anti-stroke diet may include:

- Belgian endives and celery sticks served with 1/2 cup salsa

- cherry tomatoes and broccoli florets served with 1/4 cup low-fat yogurt-based dip (try Greek yogurt with a sprinkling of salt, pepper, and garlic powder)

- carrot and celery sticks served with 1/4 cup hummus or guacamole

- 1 hard-boiled egg

- 1 cup low-sodium tomato juice or vegetable cocktail

- 1 cup steamed or boiled edamame lightly sprinkled with salt

- 1/2 avocado drizzled with lemon juice or hot sauce and seasoned with salt and pepper

- 1 slice whole grain bread topped with 2 teaspoons of peanut, almond, or cashew butter

- 5 whole grain crackers topped with 1 1/2 ounces cheddar cheese

- 5 whole grain crackers spread with 1 or 2 tablespoons of peanut, almond, or cashew butter

- 1 or 2 unsweetened rice cakes spread with 1 or 2 tablespoons of peanut, almond, or cashew butter

- Sweet snacks on the anti-stroke diet may include:

- 1 peach, pear, orange, apple, or tangerine

- 1/2 cup red grapes

- 1/2 cup fresh strawberries, blueberries, blackberries, or raspberries

- 1/2 cup blueberries and a handful of almonds

- 1 cup red grapes or blueberries, placed in a plastic bag and frozen

- 1 cup whole grain cereal with low-fat milk, berries, and a teaspoon of unprocessed honey if needed

- 1/2 toasted whole grain English muffin spread with 1 tablespoon peanut butter, thin slices of apple, and a sprinkling of cinnamon.

- 1 banana rolled in 1 1/2 ounces chopped nuts

- 1 apple and a handful of walnuts

- 1 cup plain Greek yogurt sweetened with a teaspoon of unprocessed honey or chopped fresh fruit

Nourishing snacks remind you that you don't always have to worry about putting together a whole meal. This fact is especially important for stroke patients who are recovering and may be exhausted from therapy. If a patient is too tired to make a main dish, he could simply pour some whole grain cereal or yogurt into a dish, add some berries, low-fat milk (if using cereal), nuts, and perhaps a little honey or xylitol. Or he could have cheese and whole grain crackers, carrot sticks, and a piece of fruit with a glass of tomato juice. Snacks should be simple but healthy, and the time saved in preparation may be spent taking a nap.

DINING OUT

Dining out can be fun for anyone, but it can be particularly so for a recovering stroke patient, as it gives him the chance to spend time with friends and family and enjoy delicious food that he doesn't have to prepare for himself. Unfortunately, dining out can also throw a wrench into a stroke patient's well-planned diet. Restaurants generally offer large portions of food that is loaded with salt and fat. But this fact doesn't mean a stroke patient must eat at home for every single meal in order to protect his health. Many restaurants offer satisfying choices that are nutritious and will fit into the anti-stroke diet, and many are willing to modify their offerings to accommodate customers.

> ## *Advice for Caregivers*
> ## AVOIDING THE STRESS OF DINING OUT
>
> Going out to eat can be a fun experience and a welcome change of scenery for a recovering stroke patient, but it can also be very stressful. Being surrounded by a large number of other people, dealing with the noise, and having to find appropriate seating can lead a person to feel anxious quite easily, whether he is a stroke survivor or not. If you are caring for a stroke patient and would like to take him out to eat, perhaps start with a trip to a quiet coffee shop for a short, enjoyable time. Work up to a lunch place before you try dinner. If possible, go for meals on the early side so you won't have to wait. In addition, don't dine at a place that is known to have slow service. It may be helpful to choose a place where you know the receptionist or a waitress or waiter.

Inspect the Menu Ahead of Time

Many restaurants either post their menus online or offer printed copies that you can keep on file. It is a good idea to read through a menu before visiting a restaurant to determine whether it offers any good anti-stroke choices, such as salad, salmon, or skinless chicken. Doing so will also help bring to mind any questions about ingredients or cooking methods. Some restaurants may be flexible in the way they prepare their dishes if a request is made in advance, which may be done over the phone. Choosing the right restaurant greatly improves the chances of sticking to the anti-stroke diet when dining out.

Be Smart About Portion Sizes

As recently mentioned, most restaurants offer oversized portions. The result is that many of us overload on fat, salt, and sugar every time we dine out. The following tips provide advice on how to deal with restaurant-size servings:

- Ask the server if you can order a smaller portion. Some restaurants are willing to serve a half-size portion, usually at a reduced price.

- Eat out for lunch instead of dinner. Both portions and prices are substantially smaller at lunchtime than they are at dinnertime, so you can cut down on fat, salt, and sugar while saving money in the process.

- Split an entrée with someone.

- Eat only half your meal and take the other half home.

- Create a meal out of appetizers and side dishes, such as a cup of vegetable soup, a shrimp cocktail, and a salad.

- Request generous portions of vegetables and small portions of meat.

- Swap out unhealthy sides (e.g., French fries, macaroni and cheese, mashed potatoes, etc.) for healthy ones (e.g., salad, fruit, etc.).

Choose the Way a Dish Is Prepared

Unless a restaurant prohibits any substitutions, you will probably be able to get many meals prepared the way you wish. For instance, if a restaurant offers fish that's breaded and fried, ask for the fish to be poached or grilled instead. Request that French fries be replaced with grilled tomatoes, green salad, or a side of steamed veggies. A white potato with the skin is also a good substitute and can be topped with a little butter or a small spoonful of sour cream. Salad can be served with dressing on the side, and a salad's iceberg lettuce can be replaced with mixed greens, romaine lettuce, or perhaps spinach, each of which is more nutritious than iceberg lettuce.

If a restaurant has any whole grain bread on hand, it should replace white bread on the plate. Instead of butter for the bread, olive oil can be used for dipping. If food has not been pre-seasoned, it can be prepared with only a small amount of salt or with no salt at all. Dishes can also be prepared with olive oil instead of butter. Ordering fish or poultry is a healthier choice than ordering beef or pork, but if

FOLLOWING A HEALTHY DIET
IN AN ASSISTED LIVING FACILITY

If a stroke patient lives in a facility where meals are planned and pre-pared by others, he can still choose wholesome foods and follow other lifestyle habits that support good brain and heart health. Often menus are brought around for the next day, giving him a chance to check the healthiest items offered. If a dietitian comes around from time to time, a stroke patient or his loved one could discuss the types of foods he'd like to see on the menu and the ways he would like to have his meals prepared. If foods are served buffet-style in a community dining room, he could choose a couple of servings of fruits and vegetables at every meal, including breakfast. He could also ask for poached, soft-boiled, or hard-boiled eggs; and select fish, poultry, and—less frequently—lean beef or pork. Dessert shouldn't be a regular part of a meal, but when it is requested, fresh fruit, low-fat yogurt, or low-fat frozen yogurt would be the best choices.

When family and friends visit assisted living facilities, they tend to bring unhealthy snacks like cookies, candies, or cake. A patient can ask them to bring fresh fruits and unsalted nuts, unsalted popcorn, or whole grain crackers instead. The facility should also be advised to provide healthy snacks.

A patient may wish to take nutritional supplements to fill in gaps in his diet, but a facility may be concerned about possible interactions between his supplements and any medication he is taking, so his health-care provider will need to make the final decision on this issue.

beef or pork is part of a meal, it should be the smallest, leanest piece available and served with veggies such as cooked carrots, asparagus, broccoli, string beans, Brussels sprouts, baked potatoes, or a large salad. Due to their high calorie counts, creamy sauces and cheese toppings should be avoided or placed on the side so only a small amount is used.

Anyone who is trying to protect or improve their health should stay away from fast food restaurants, as they are known for their high-fat, high-sodium fare. If a person on a healthy diet finds himself at a fast food restaurant, he should look at all the options available and, if possible, choose a green salad, grilled chicken, yogurt, or some other wholesome choice. If several burgers are on the menu and he is determined to have one, he should choose the smallest one—no bigger than four ounces (about the size of a deck of cards).

Skip or Downsize Dessert

It is perfectly reasonable to skip dessert and enjoy a cup of tea or coffee instead. Many of us are no longer even hungry by the time we reach the dessert portion of a restaurant meal. If, however, the craving for something sweet at the end of a meal is present, a restaurant should be able to provide fruit—either fresh or poached—or a serving of sorbet. If a piece of cake or pie must be had, it could always be shared with others at the table.

CONCLUSION

The anti-stroke diet can be followed at home, when dining out, and when living in an assisted living facility because there's nothing exotic, unusual, or particularly difficult about this meal plan. As long as an individual maintains a high intake of vegetables, legumes, fruits, nuts, unrefined cereals, and olive oil; a moderate intake of fish; a low to moderate intake of dairy products (mostly in the form of cheese or yogurt); and a low intake of saturated fat, meat, and poultry, that individual will be eating well and using nutrition to lower his chance of stroke.

PART IV

Life after a Stroke

14

$\mathscr{D}$ealing with the Stroke Effects You Cannot See

$\mathbf{P}$revious chapters have dealt with obvious effects of stroke—weakness, balance difficulties, poor coordination, and vision and language issues. This chapter addresses common stroke effects you cannot see: depression, anxiety, pain, sleep problems, and fatigue. These issues can worsen quality of life and slow improvement of physical symptoms. Managing these conditions will optimize recovery.

We have all experienced certain negative emotions or feelings at times in our lives, but they are usually mild, temporary, and easily improved. We may experience sadness, despair, or irritability after events in our lives, such as a difficult divorce, a move, job loss, or the death of a family member, friend, or beloved pet. These feelings, though intense, are usually temporary, and improve with time, allowing us to bounce back. Depression is different. It's likely caused by chemical changes in the brain, and one cannot just "snap out of it."

Similarly, most of us have experienced anxiety at times—before an important speech or performance, walking into an exam, heading to a job interview, or awaiting surgery. Who hasn't experienced fatigue after a physically or mentally stressful event, such as a long run, a tennis match, working in the yard, filling out taxes, or a sleepless night? But rest and a good night's sleep usually relieve this exhaustion. Anxiety and fatigue after stroke can last longer.

At one time or another, we have all experienced different types of pain, whether from root canals, broken bones, or pain after surgery.

These improve and disappear given time, and pain medications can be helpful in the short term. Other pain occurs repeatedly or chronically—like sinus headaches, migraines, or arthritis. Pain after stroke can be due to various causes: tightness in muscles (spasticity), misalignment of the shoulder joint in the setting of arm weakness (shoulder subluxation), or, rarely, abnormal signals from the part of the brain that perceives pain, known as the thalamus.

Advice for Caregivers
ADJUSTING TO YOUR NEW LOVED ONE

Depression, anxiety, fatigue, pain, and sleep problems are common after stroke. If you are the caregiver of a loved one who has had a stroke, these conditions may be as distressing to you as they are to him. It's important for you to understand what your loved one may be going through. By discussing the questions found in the relevant sections of this chapter with your loved one, you should achieve a better understanding of how he is feeling. The answers you both reach together through this conversation may be shared with his doctor, physician assistant, nurse practitioner, nurses, social worker, or therapists.

Try not to minimize his situation. If he is depressed, there is no point in telling him to cheer up or count his blessings, or to point out how much worse things could be. He may not be able to articulate why he feels depressed. If he is overly anxious, don't tell him not to be such a "worrywart." If he suffers from severe fatigue, don't tell him he simply needs to try harder, or not to be a "lazybones." Be sensitive to his situation and treat him as you would want to be treated if the situation were reversed. Be patient and kind, and consult the treatments and tips recommended in this chapter to help him.

Most of us have problems with sleep from time to time. We can't fall asleep, or we wake up in the middle of the night and are unable to get back to sleep, or we wake up too early and toss and turn until it is time to get up. Usually, these problems improve with time and resolve themselves. Sometimes medication is needed temporarily. The depression, anxiety, fatigue, pain, and sleep problems that may result from a stroke, however, are different from similar issues that may occur as a consequence of typical daily life. They may be mild, but they may also be severe or crippling. They may not improve quickly, tending to drag on and on. They are often overlooked and go untreated.

DEPRESSION

Depression is common after a stroke, affecting approximately one-third of stroke survivors at any one time after stroke (compared with 5 to 13 percent of adults without stroke). There are numerous potential reasons for depression after stroke, including psychological reactions to having cognitive and functional impairments, as well as changes in the brain (including altered levels of neurotransmitters, disruption of nerve networks, and inflammation). Risk factors for depression after stroke include physical disability, cognitive impairment, and severity of stroke (the more severe the stroke, the higher the association with depression afterwards).

Depression is associated with worse functional outcomes. This means that people with untreated depression are less likely to recover from their strokes. For this reason, it is critical to spot the warning signs of depression and start treating it right away. In fact, one trial that looked at the use of an antidepressant, fluoxetine, on movement and strength after stroke found that those who took fluoxetine experienced better recoveries after stroke.

Depression doesn't mean just having the blues or feeling down. Such reactions are typical after a stroke. In order to identify symptoms of depression in a stroke patient, use the acronym "SIGECAPS" as a mnemonic device. "S" stands for sleep: Does he have insomnia or does he oversleep? "I" stands for interest: Does he have less interest in things that used to excite him? "G" stands for guilt: Does he feel guilty or feel like he has let himself or his family down? "E" stands for energy: Does he feel tired or have little energy? "C" stands for concentration: Does he have difficulty concentrating, reading the newspaper, or watching television? "A" stands for appetite: Does he have a poor appetite or does he overeat? "P" stands for psychomotor retardation, which is a scientific term for moving and talking slowly: Does he move or speak so slowly that other people have noticed? The final letter "S" stands for suicide: Does he feel hopeless and have suicidal thoughts?

Obviously, some of these symptoms may be effects of the stroke, unrelated to depression. For example, a stroke patient may move slowly due to weakness or have difficulty concentrating due to the cognitive effects of stroke. It is therefore important to talk to a health-care provider so she can screen for depression and use her expertise to make a diagnosis.

Depression Management

Managing depression can include making lifestyle changes, receiving counseling and psychotherapeutic treatments, taking medication, and trying complementary therapies. Often a multipronged and holistic approach that incorporates each of these elements proves most effective. There are several key lifestyle changes that can help manage depression, such as eating a healthy diet, engaging in regular physical activity, limiting or avoiding alcohol and drug use, keeping a regimented sleep schedule, and meditating. The good news is that most of these factors also help reduce the risk of another stroke.

As you might have guessed, what you eat can affect your moods. Eating red meat or processed meat, refined grains, or sweets can increase a person's risk of depression. Diets low in fruits and vegetables also elevate this risk. Eating unhealthy foods while trying to recover from a stroke is like delivering the wrong materials to a bicycle factory and expecting the bicycles it manufactures to work properly. They simply won't, and the factory will have to be shut down. If the brain and body do not get what they need, they will not function optimally, and depression will linger. Stroke patients should eat foods with nutrients that will help their brains work better, such as fruits and vegetables, whole grains, fish, legumes, nuts, and healthy fats.

In the case of vitamin deficiency, dietary supplements may be helpful in reducing the risk of depression, but there is little scientific evidence of this effect in connection with stroke patients. In fact, few randomized clinical trials have assessed the impact of vitamin supplementation on depression after stroke. A few studies have examined *associations* between vitamin levels and depression after stroke. Keep in mind that just because a certain vitamin or mineral deficiency may be linked to depression after stroke, it does not mean that giving patients that vitamin or mineral will reduce the risk of depression after stroke. That question may be answered only with a double-blind, randomized clinical trial in which one group gets the vitamin, the other group (which is comparable with respect to characteristics such as age, gender, and stroke severity) gets a placebo (sugar pill), and neither the patients nor the people running the trial know which group is getting what (i.e., they are both "blinded") until after the assessments are done. That being said, we will discuss a few possible associations between vitamin deficiencies and depression after stroke.

Low levels of magnesium after stroke have been related to depression at three months after a stroke. In a very small study (sixty patients), when studied in depressed patients (although not stroke survivors) with low blood magnesium, daily magnesium supplements taken for eight or more weeks improved depression and increased blood magnesium. Larger trials in stroke survivors are needed to determine if magnesium supplementation in those with low magnesium is helpful in reducing depression symptoms after stroke. Stroke patients can ask their healthcare providers to measure their magnesium levels. If they come back as low, a supplement of 250 mg to 500 mg of magnesium oxide each day may be beneficial.

B vitamins have been studied extensively in stroke survivors because they are involved in the metabolism of the amino acid homocysteine, high levels of which have been associated with stroke. In one study that looked at the effect of B vitamins on depression after stroke, stroke survivors who were followed for an average of seven years and had taken daily vitamin B_9 (folic acid) (2 mg), vitamin B_6 (25 mg), and vitamin B_{12} (0.5 mg) during this time displayed a lower risk of developing depression than those who had not. A point to keep in mind is that over 99 percent of individuals in this trial were living in countries that do not add folate to cereal grains. In the United States and Canada, cereal grain products have added folic acid. This public health intervention was implemented to reduce the likelihood of children being born with neural tube defects (folate is essential during pregnancy for neural tube development). Therefore, the effect of B vitamin supplementation on depression in stroke survivors who live in countries that add folic acid to grains is unknown. Another important point is that this trial had follow-up information for only half its participants. (Only 273 participants were able to be followed until the final assessment.)

Low blood levels of vitamin D have been linked to depression after stroke—levels of vitamin D at admission were associated with depression at one month. No clinical trials, however, have tested whether taking vitamin D supplements reduces risk of depression after stroke. If a stroke patient's level of vitamin D is low, he may need to take a vitamin D supplement, as diet is not a great source of this nutrient. Sunshine activates production of vitamin D in the body, but, of course, sunscreen use, which is highly recommended to prevent skin cancer, hinders this process. Given the scant evidence of vitamin supplements improving depression after stroke, it is important to eat a healthy diet, which provides all the necessary nutrients and vitamins.

Five trials of psychological therapy (enrolling 521 participants) showed a 23 percent reduction in depression relapses and recurrences in those receiving psychotherapy. These studies were also variable, making comparisons difficult.

Of course, depression often cannot be managed solely with lifestyle changes, counseling, or psychotherapeutic treatments, in which case there are numerous medications available that may help. The medications most frequently studied in clinical trials of stroke patients are selective serotonin reuptake inhibitors, or SSRIs. (See page 130.) The pooled results of eight trials of medication interventions after stroke (enrolling a total of 1,025 participants) showed that medications were associated with a 30 percent reduction in depression relapses and recurrence. Unfortunately, there was a great deal of variability in these trials, so it is difficult to compare them. Additionally, most did not treat patients for an adequate period of time.

Several complementary therapies, including acupressure, massage, and aromatherapy, may also help reduce depression. (See Chapter 8 on page 114 for discussions on each.)

ANXIETY

Anxiety is actually the most common mental health issue across the board, with up to 30 percent of individuals developing anxiety over the course of their lifetime. Among stroke survivors, anxiety is common. Up to 30 percent of stroke survivors develop anxiety in the first year after stroke.

From a psychological perspective, anxiety is described as a type of fear or worry. When a person is anxious, he can experience physical sensations and discomfort such as chest tightness or restlessness. When anxiety is mild, a person can feel worried or troubled. When it is severe, he may experience fear or panic. If a person was anxious before his stroke, he is more likely to experience increased anxiety after his stroke.

Anxiety is a normal part of everyday life. So, when do you know if someone has an anxiety disorder? In order for it to be classified as a disorder, it must cause significant distress or impairment in a person's social relationships, job performance, or other important areas of his life.

After a stroke, concerns and anxiety can be expected. Stroke survivors often worry about having another stroke, not recovering from a stroke, not being able to take care of themselves and their families, and being unable to return to work. So, how do you know if anxiety is a normal reaction to stroke or is more troublesome? It can help to take an anxiety survey to see how severe the symptoms are. (See Table 14.1 on the following page.) In addition, it's incredibly important to discuss your symptoms with a healthcare provider.

Anxiety Management

Management options for anxiety include relaxation techniques (e.g., meditation), lifestyle changes (e.g., regular sleep, healthy diet, abstaining from drugs and alcohol), psychotherapy, and medication. We still don't know the optimal management strategy for anxiety after stroke, as we don't have enough large high-quality randomized clinical trials of stroke survivors. However, in the meantime, it makes sense to manage anxiety after stroke similarly to the way in which anxiety is managed in individuals who have not had a stroke.

TABLE 14.1. GENERALIZED ANXIETY DISORDER (GAD-7)

(Circle the number to indicate your answer.)

Over the last two weeks, how often have you been bothered by the following problems?	Not at all	Several days	More than half the days	Every day
1. Feeling nervous, anxious, or on edge	0	1	2	3
2. Not being able to stop or control worrying	0	1	2	3
3. Worrying too much about different things	0	1	2	3
4. Trouble relaxing	0	1	2	3
5. Being so restless that it's hard to sit still	0	1	2	3
6. Becoming easily annoyed or irritated	0	1	2	3
7. Feeling afraid as if something awful might happen	0	1	2	3
Add the Score for Each Column	+____	+____	+____	+____
Add Your Column Scores for Total Score =				

A score of 5 or less indicates mild anxiety; a score of 6 to 10 points to moderate anxiety; and a score of 10 or greater suggests severe anxiety. Anxious patients should show this questionnaire to their health-care providers.

Relaxation techniques are particularly effective in managing anxiety. In addition, several complementary therapies can be helpful, including tai chi and yoga, which are calming. Acupuncture and acupressure may also improve anxiety, while massage therapy is known to reduce stress. Music therapy can also be soothing, and aromatherapy—lavender, for instance—may relieve stress. Just as it can mitigate depression, a very nutritious diet may also ease anxiety. Regular physical activity can also help decrease anxiety and increase mental and physical well-being.

A stroke patient who is dealing with anxiety may find relief simply in knowing he can lower his chances of having another stroke by modifying his diet, getting exercise, stopping smoking, lowering his blood pressure, etc. Just feeling like he has some degree of control over his future is bound to make him feel less anxious.

Cognitive behavioral therapy (CBT) is an effective technique in managing anxiety. It is a practical solution-oriented therapy that is aimed at examining how thoughts are connected to feelings. It seeks to alter certain thought processes in order to reduce unpleasant feelings. CBT focuses on examining a person's beliefs, thoughts, and attitudes to show how these thought processes affect how one feels. CBT aims to identify harmful thoughts, fact-check them to see if they are an accurate perception of reality, and, if they are not, employ techniques to overcome them. CBT provides patients with effective strategies for changing thought patterns. These include learning to recognize distorted thoughts and reevaluate them in light of reality; gaining a better understanding of others' behavior; using problem-solving skills; and developing confidence in one's own abilities (i.e., self-efficacy). With enough practice, patients can become skilled in managing their own thoughts and feelings, through using the practical skills learned through CBT. CBT can be done one on one or in a group setting. Sometimes group sessions provide the added benefit of social support and additional problem-solving with individuals with similar issues. In a typical CBT session, a therapist asks a client to describe specific problems and set goals to work towards. These problems and goals guide the sessions. A therapist will often assign homework to a client to help him achieve his goals. CBT is also an effective method to reduce depression.

Of course, there are medications that can relieve anxiety. Many medications used in treating depression are also used to treat anxiety, such as SSRIs. Some medications can also increase fatigue, so stroke survivors should be sure to mention fatigue when discussing their anxiety.

PAIN

Chronic pain affects about half of stroke survivors. There are numerous potential reasons for pain after stroke, including spasticity (continuous contraction of weak muscles, causing stiffness and tightness), muscle spasms (sudden contractions of muscles), contractures (shortening and hardening of muscles, limiting range of motion), shoulder pain (from subluxation, rotator cuff tears, tendinitis, or nerve impingement), neuropathic pain (from strokes affecting the part of the brain that perceives sensation), and headaches. Neuropathic pain is due to nerve damage and can cause burning, searing, or shooting pain. Neuropathic pain occurs when nerve fibers themselves are damaged, dysfunctional, or injured. It can also occur when there is a stroke in the part of the brain that receives pain signals.

Pain often goes undiagnosed and untreated. When a healthcare provider asks a stroke patient about the presence and location of any pain, it is always easier if he can understand and participate in the conversation. If a patient understands but cannot speak clearly, he can point to where it hurts and use a pain scale (see Figure 14.1 below) to identify his level of pain. A pain scale typically grades pain levels from 0 to 10, where 0 refers to no pain and 10 refers to the worst pain imaginable. Sometimes a pain scale will include pictures of different facial expressions, each of which corresponds to a degree of pain. This visual element can make it easier for a patient to determine the intensity of his pain.

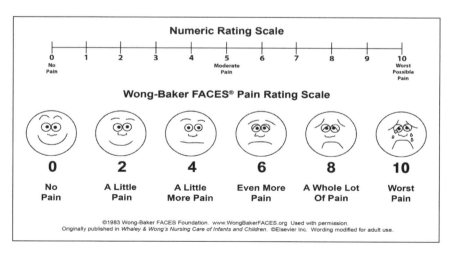

Figure 14.1. Pain Rating Scale

A stroke patient's healthcare provider needs to know if he is in pain, where this pain is located, and how severe it is so it can be treated properly.

Pain Management

Treatment of pain depends on the underlying cause. Spasticity can be treated with medication taken by mouth (such as baclofen) or injections into the muscle (such as botulinum toxin). These medications cause muscle relaxation. Contractures can be treated with physical and occupational therapy. Typically, physical and occupational therapists will use gentle stretching exercises to improve range of motion. Functional electrical stimulation can also be used to treat a painful or stiff joint. Shoulder pain can be treated with physical and occupational therapy as well as anti-inflammatory medications. Headaches are typically managed with medications such as amitriptyline or topiramate, which prevent headaches. Neuropathic pain can be managed with special medications for neuropathic pain, which include gabapentin and pregabalin. Opiates are almost never used to treat stroke patients. They are highly addictive, do not treat the underlying cause, and are not appropriate for long-term use.

SLEEP PROBLEMS

Sleep disturbances are extremely common after a stroke—about three-quarters of stroke survivors experience them. Sufficient high-quality sleep is critical for normal mental and physical health. During sleep, the brain performs "house cleaning" tasks, so to speak, disposing of harmful waste products that accumulate during waking hours. In addition, proper sleep supports a person's abilities to learn and pay attention the next day. During sleep, the brain also works on building memories and helps both the body repair itself—including the brain. Studies have also shown that sleep is important for neuroplasticity (i.e., developing new nerve networks in the brain), and can help with motor recovery after stroke. So, while decent sleep is important to everyone, it is especially important to stroke survivors.

Stroke patients may have trouble getting to sleep, staying asleep, or waking up too early. Although it is fairly obvious to identify sleep problems, a sleep questionnaire can be a valuable tool in determining the presence of an actual sleep disorder, such as sleep apnea. A healthcare provider can use a sleep questionnaire to diagnose a sleep disorder, which will help her decide how to treat it most effectively. Sleep questionnaires typically assess a patient's quality of sleep by asking a patient to gauge (on a scale of 0 to 3, for example) how often he experiences sleep problems such as waking up in the middle of the night, coughing or snoring loudly, having bad dreams, having to get up to use the bathroom, and others. His total score gives his healthcare provider a decent picture of how well (or poorly) he has been sleeping.

Sleep Management

Effective stroke recovery depends on good quality sleep—about seven to eight hours of it each night. Each person is different, though, and some may need a little more or a little less than this amount. A stroke patient may need extra sleep after experiencing a stroke. Good "sleep hygiene," which refers to good sleep habits that can lead to a better night's sleep, is important for everyone to maintain, but particularly for stroke patients. (See inset on page 247.)

Pain relief is obviously important if pain is preventing a restful night. (See page 242.) In addition, heavy meals should be avoided at least four hours before bedtime, and a healthy diet should be followed in general. (See Chapter 13 on page 215.) If a snack is desired before bedtime, complex carbohydrates such as whole grain bread or cereal; lean protein such as nut butter, low-fat cheese, chicken, turkey, or fish; or a beverage such as warm milk or chamomile tea can satisfy the urge without straying from the anti-stroke eating plan. Foods with simple carbohydrates, added sugar, or high salt contents, such as white bread, ice cream, or chips, should be avoided. Caffeinated beverages should not be consumed after dinner. Decaf coffee or tea is fine. Stroke patients who are very sensitive to caffeine should not have any caffeinated drink after 2 PM.

If a patient's sleep does not improve through lifestyle choices and sleep hygiene, his healthcare provider may recommend medication, but this is generally discouraged after a stroke. Instead of reaching for her prescription pad, however, she may recommend a calming tea, such as valerian or kava tea. Some research has shown that these teas can decrease sleep onset time and promote deeper sleep. She may also recommend alternative calming practices such as tai chi, acupuncture, yoga, or meditation. (See pages 116 to 121.)

FATIGUE

Fatigue is common after stroke—up to 70 percent of survivors experience it—and it may be one of the most distressing symptoms. It's helpful to understand that fatigue is common and will improve. One way to think about it is to think about the brain's energy needs.

The brain needs a lot of energy—20 percent of total energy—to work. After a stroke, a survivor's brain requires even more energy in order to heal, which makes him feel exhausted. In addition, strokes in certain areas of the brain can cause sleepiness. For example, the brainstem contains nerve fibers that maintain alertness. If a stroke impacts both sides of the brainstem, stroke patients can be quite sleepy, particularly in the first few days after a stroke. Another area associated with sleepiness is the thalamus. In addition, if a stroke is large and causes brain swelling, the stroke survivor can be sleepy in the first few days.

Other things that can cause fatigue are lack of sleep, infection (such as pneumonia or urinary tract infection), and metabolic abnormalities caused by liver or kidney problems. While fatigue is common after stroke, severe sleepiness can be a sign of a complication such as brain swelling or bleeding. If you are the caregiver of a stroke survivor and cannot wake him up, even with repeated tactile stimulation (such as tapping or shaking him), call 911.

Fatigue Management

When it comes to reducing fatigue, several things can help: good sleep hygiene (see inset on page 247), a healthy diet, regular exercise (without overdoing it), depression treatment, adjusting medications that cause sleepiness, and complementary therapies such as tai chi, yoga, and massage. As sleep problems (see page 244), which can lead to fatigue, are present in more than half of stroke survivors, any stroke patient who struggles to get to sleep or stay asleep, or who wakes up too early, should mention these problems to his healthcare provider so she can help him alleviate them. Resting during the day may help with fatigue, as long as these rest periods don't disrupt nighttime sleep. (For other ways to improve sleep, see page 245.)

The body depends upon the diet for its energy needs. When fatigue sets in, it is very easy to reach for salty or sweet snacks and sugary beverages, which will temporarily decrease fatigue but do nothing to help the brain or body to heal and feel better. A better choice would be fruit, vegetables, whole grains, lean meat, nuts, legumes, or milk.

GOOD SLEEP HYGIENE

Good sleep hygiene involves following this expert advice:

- Go to bed at the same time every night—including weekends and holidays—and get up at the same time every morning. Doing so will "set" your built-in "sleep clock."

- Get at least seven hours of sleep each night.

- Don't go to bed unless you are sleepy.

- If you don't fall asleep after 20 minutes, get out of bed.

- Establish a routine for the hour before bedtime. Before this hour arrives, make a list of all the things you need to do the next day and then forget about them. Make the hour before bedtime a quiet, peaceful time. You may want to take a warm, relaxing bath—if you are able to navigate a bathtub safely. You may enjoy reading (but not in bed, and nothing upsetting), listening to soft music, meditating, praying, or simply thinking about the good things that happened that day.

- Keep your room at a comfortable, cool temperature—60°F to 70°F. Have a blanket at the bottom of your bed to pull up if you get chilly.

- Avoid daytime naps.

- Make sure you are exposed to natural light during the day.

- Exercise daily for as long as you are able—until you are tired but not exhausted. Exercising outside is best because sunlight helps set your sleep-wake cycle. Try not to exercise within three hours of bedtime, as exercise can be stimulating.

- Do not use alcohol as a sleep aid. While alcohol may help you feel sleepy, it reduces the quality of your sleep. You may find you wake in the middle of the night and are unable to get back to sleep.

- Break your nicotine habit if you have one. Nicotine is a stimulant and can cause sleep problems.

- Avoid electronics for at least two hours before bed. This includes the TV, computer, and smartphone.

- Don't fall asleep listening to the TV or radio. Your room should also be free of noise. If your partner snores, you may want to use ear plugs or a "white noise" machine, such as a fan or humidifier.

- Do not eat, watch TV, read, or work in bed. Your bed is to be used only for sleep (and sex if you have a partner).

- Keep your room dark at night and in the early morning. Use black-out curtains or eye shades. Use a motion-detection night light so you won't fall if you get up to go to the bathroom in the middle of the night.

- Use comfortable and supportive pillows.

Mild exercise may alleviate fatigue—a benefit stroke patients will truly appreciate—but survivors should make a point not to overdo it when exercising. They should start slowly and see if they can increase the pace a little each day, building up strength and stamina. In general, it's important for stroke patients to pace themselves, listen to their bodies, and allow themselves plenty of time to get dressed and ready to exercise, as they may require more time to do these things than they did before their strokes. Physical or occupational therapy should be scheduled on different days than exercise.

Since depression can sap a patient of his energy, treating depression—whether through lifestyle changes (healthy diet, physical activity, and abstaining from drug and alcohol use), counseling, or psychotherapeutic treatments—may also mean improving fatigue.

Certain medications prescribed after a stroke may make a patient more tired than usual. This problem may be solved by lowering the dosage or replacing the fatigue-related medication with one that doesn't cause fatigue. Perhaps the timing of a drug's administration should be adjusted. Whatever the answer may be, a healthcare provider should be consulted before a stroke survivor makes any changes to his medication regimen.

Complementary therapies such tai chi or yoga can help reduce fatigue, and because these activities are slower and gentler than typical exercise regimens, they may suit a greater number of stroke patients. Massage can reduce stress and anxiety, and therefore the fatigue that can accompany these states. Aromatherapy may also be helpful.

CONCLUSION

Depression, anxiety, pain, sleep problems, and fatigue are all common issues after a stroke. They can cause frustration, interfere with recovery, and decrease quality of life. Fortunately, all these issues can improve with a healthy diet, regular physical activity, and sleep hygiene. In addition, since these conditions are often related to each other, improvement in one can lessen the severity of another condition. For example, if a patient alleviates his depression, his fatigue and pain may also dissipate considerably, allowing him to participate more in therapies such as OT and PT, which will aid in his recovery. In some cases, medication can be helpful in treating these problems. In other cases, the simple lifestyle changes recommended in this chapter may be all that is needed.

15

$\mathscr{L}$iving Successfully after a Stroke

Previous chapters of this book have explained what strokes are, how to decrease the risk of having a first stroke or recurrent strokes, and how to optimize recovery from a stroke. This chapter provides advice on how to live successfully after coming home from a hospital unit, rehabilitation center, or skilled nursing facility.

Most stroke survivors are not able to waltz back into their old lives, even if they seem to be doing well. Everything will require more thought and planning. No matter how simple a task may be, it will likely take more time to accomplish. Whether it is due to newfound difficulties in getting dressed in the morning, preparing a simple meal, or going grocery shopping, frustration can easily set in. Every stroke survivor should keep in mind that this reaction is perfectly normal.

Most stroke patients have much less energy after their strokes. Daily chores can make them physically and mentally exhausted in ways they never had before, but this exhaustion generally improves over time. If a patient feels the need to rest, he should go right ahead. Doing so will actually help his brain to rewire itself and recover from injury. Recognizing his low energy level, he will need to ration his available energy so that he is able to get his most important tasks accomplished. In light of this fact, picking up medications, preparing easy heart- and brain-healthy meals and snacks, going to therapy, and going to healthcare provider appointments should be at the top of his to-do list.

It's reasonable to assume that every house or apartment will have its own set of challenges for a person with physical limitations caused by a stroke. After a stroke, a survivor's living space may seem full of obstacles in the way of successful everyday routines. While there is no one answer that can solve every problem, there are a number of ways to minimize the difficulties a stroke patient may find when getting back to his life at home. This chapter provides many practical suggestions to create a living environment that is as safe and comfortable as possible for a stroke survivor.

LIVING SAFELY

When a stroke survivor is deemed ready to return home, one of the therapists from the hospital or rehabilitation center will likely talk to him and his loved ones about making his home safe. A physical or occupational therapist may even visit his home to see what potential barriers may exist. Often, the therapist will tour the home with the stroke survivor's loved ones or primary caregiver. The therapist will point out dangerous areas and make suggestions that will turn a possibly hazardous situation into a safer one.

Falls are common in anyone over the age of sixty-five and are therefore considered a major public health problem. Not surprisingly, they are even more common in stroke survivors. A fall may be due to low blood sugar or low blood pressure, or it may be caused by a stroke's effects on balance, vision, coordination, or strength.

This section offers methods to avoid some of the most common problems a survivor may face in his living space.

Entrance

Therapists will address all the issues involved in getting into a living space, from getting out of a vehicle to actually entering a home. Will a patient be able to walk securely from his car to his front door? Will he be able to use his key to enter his house? Will he need to climb steps? Is there a railing, and if not, can one be installed? (A patient can practice walking up and down stairs in therapy, too.) If he enters through the garage, are there steps? Installing a simple railing for these steps could be important. If he is using a wheelchair, a ramp may need to be installed.

Clutter and Lighting

It is important to remove any items a stroke survivor could trip over in the home and tidy up any clutter could cause a fall. For example, it is very easy to trip over an area rug. Area rugs should be removed. The same goes for certain pieces of furniture such as footstools. In addition, rooms and halls should be well lit. A patient may need more night lights, which may be motion-activated.

Kitchen

In a stroke survivor's kitchen, is there a chair for him to sit down if he gets tired? Are items such as pots and pans and other kitchen utensils easily accessible? What about dishes, glasses, and silverware? Are healthy foods located on shelves he can easily reach? (They shouldn't be placed on too high a shelf, as looking up may cause a loss of balance.) It is important to note that using a microwave may be safer than using a stove or oven after a stroke. Of course, if there are any small rugs or mats in the kitchen, they should be removed.

Advice for Caregivers
MAKING A HOUSE OR APARTMENT SAFE

If one of your loved one's therapists recommends a home visit, take a notebook and join her so you can make notes of any needed changes, which may be as simple as removing area rugs or objects your loved one could trip over. You may need to buy some nightlights so that he won't fall when getting up at night. You may need to buy a shower chair. Or the changes may be more complicated, such as putting up railings next to steps or installing grab bars in the bathroom. If you don't have the time or skills required to do these things, find a handyperson who can makes these changes for you. Be ready to ask your loved one's therapist questions about any concerns you may have. Following the therapist's recommendations will lower your loved one's risk of falling or tripping.

Bedroom and Bathroom

Moving on to the bedroom and bathroom, are there area rugs that need to be removed? Are clothes easily accessible in a well-lit closet or in a chest of drawers? Are there night lights in both the bedroom and bathroom? An easily reached overhead light or bedside lamp may also be helpful.

Bathrooms can be dangerous places—perhaps the most dangerous place in the house. Bathmats are extremely easy to trip over, and a bathroom floor makes for a very hard landing after a fall. Most accidents occur near the shower, bathtub, or toilet. In light of this fact, a urinal or potty chair placed by the bedside may be easier and safer to use than walking to the bathroom at night. It is worth noting that more falls occur when a person is getting out of a shower or tub than getting into one, probably because the floor of the tub or shower is slippery from the soap and water at that point. Everyone, especially stroke survivors, should put non-slip strips on their tub or shower floors—and around their tubs or showers if need be. Slippery floors should be avoided at all costs.

Having grab bars installed can greatly increase the safety of a bathroom. A physical or occupational therapist can explain exactly where they would need to be placed for maximum safety. Putting benches or chairs in a shower can be helpful if a stroke survivor suddenly gets tired or feels off-balance and needs to sit down to bathe. Changing his shower head so he can hold it in his hand may make things easier, too. Finally, a special elevated toilet seat may help him sit and stand more easily when he needs to use the toilet.

Stairs

Are there stairs in the house? If so, are there banisters or railings to hold on to? If not, it would be a good idea to install them. Are the stairs well lit? Are there especially steep stairs in the house that should be avoided, such as those going down to the basement? Whatever is down there is not worth a hip or skull fracture. Along these lines, a person who has experienced a stroke should never climb ladders or stepstools until his therapist agrees he can do so safely.

MEDICAL ALERT SYSTEM

A medical alert system is a must for a stroke survivor. According to the Centers for Disease Control, approximately one in four adults aged sixty-five or older reports falling in a given year. Survivors are even more likely to fall due to muscle weakness, lack of balance, vision changes, medication side effects, low blood sugar, or low blood pressure.

Some people may feel that using a medical alert system means they have lost their independence, but actually, these devices support an independent lifestyle and provide peace of mind. A stroke survivor can be active inside and even outside his home, knowing that help will be available if it is needed. These devices can also be used in the event of a robbery or a fire.

So, how do medical alerts work? In most cases, a patient's home is monitored electronically by a button he wears on his wrist or around his neck. When the button is pressed, a signal is sent to a base unit, which then sends an emergency signal though to the company that is monitoring the individual. The person being monitored is then connected with a trained operator, who sends emergency help to him.

When choosing a medical alert system, a stroke patent should consider the following:

- **What does he want the system to do?** Does he simply want to be able to call for help in the event of an emergency, or does he also

ESTABLISHING A ROUTINE

Every stroke patient should set a daily routine for himself, which may help him remember to take his medications, keep his therapy sessions, go to his healthcare providers' appointments, get regular sleep, engage in regular physical activity, and prepare and eat healthy meals.

Getting the Home Organized

Getting a stroke survivor's home organized will help him plan each day successfully. In one place, he may want to have all his papers and devices he needs. This could be his favorite armchair in his living want daily check-ins and other services? Different companies offer different programs. If he falls, would his system detect this event and call automatically for help?

- **What type of equipment would work best for him?** Is the device comfortable to wear, and does it show? Is it waterproof and therefore able to be worn in the shower or bath (which is very important)? What are its range, mobility, and connectivity? Does it include GPS so that it will protect him anywhere he goes?

- **How quickly will the company respond, and who will respond?** Ideally, the response time should be seconds, not minutes, and he should be able to talk to a live person who is available 24/7.

- **What does the system cost?** A potential customer should look for a company with no extra fees for equipment, shipping, installation, activation, or service and repair. He should pay only ongoing monthly fees and avoid entering into a long-term contract.

Once a patient chooses a system, he should practice using it to see how it works for him. If it's not a good fit, he should switch to a company that can provide the practical protection and peace of mind he needs. Once he has settled on a monitoring company and gets his button, he should never take it off.

room or family room, with a table next to his chair—perhaps one with drawers and extra shelves—and another table or couch on the other side. If he has difficulty getting out of a chair, purchasing a chair that lifts him up to stand may be a good idea. His cell or landline phone and his TV remote should be kept in this special spot. Here are some other things to keep there:

- Phone numbers of healthcare providers, pharmacies, rehabilitation center, friends, and family

- File folder with all discharge instructions from the hospital or rehabilitation facility and from outpatient rehabilitation

- Pencil, paper or a notebook, and perhaps scissors

- Appointment book and calendar

- Newspaper, books, magazines, puzzle books, and TV remote

While it is nice to have all the things he frequently needs next to him, it's also important for a stroke patient to get up and move around as often and as much as he is able. As the old saying goes, "If you don't use it, you'll lose it."

Advice for Caregivers
LEARNING ABOUT MEDICATIONS

It is extremely important for a stroke patient to take the medicines he has been prescribed exactly as directed by his healthcare provider. When your loved one is discharged, be sure you and he understand all his healthcare provider's recommendations. Ask her questions. If necessary, ask her to repeat instructions. Ask why each drug has been prescribed. Ask her to explain further if you don't understand something. Ask her if there are any likely side effects. Have her call in prescriptions to your pharmacy so they will be ready for pick-up or perhaps delivered to his house.

Be sure both you and your loved one set up a system so he won't forget to take his pills. A pill organizer can be extremely helpful. It's also helpful to put a sticker on each pill bottle that indicates what the medication is for. Make sure he understands how important these medications are. If he appears to be experiencing any side effects, immediately call his healthcare provider's office and speak with her or her nurse about them. Try to minimize unnecessary medications. For example, if he was prescribed a stool softener in the hospital, does he need it now?

Taking Medications

We cannot emphasize enough how important it is for a stroke patient to take all his medications every day and at the right time. After being discharged from a hospital or rehabilitation facility, a survivor must understand which medications to take and when to take them. Medical staff will provide both verbal and written instructions. A family member or friend should also understand his prescriptions and why he needs to take them.

If picking up prescriptions and refills from the pharmacy is a problem, some pharmacies and insurance plans deliver. There are also mail-order pharmacies that deliver to the home, but this type of service may cause a delay at first. (In the meantime, he may need to use his local pharmacy.) Patients should mark on their calendars the dates when they will need to reorder medications. Remember that each pill bottle will have the number of refills left on a prescription marked on its label. When that number is 0, a refill should be requested.

In order to keep track of medications and reduce the chances of missing or forgetting to take medications, organization is the key. There are several ways to organize medications, but one of the most effective is to use a pill organizer. A pill organizer is a plastic container with little boxes relegated to each day of the week and different times of the day. These containers come in different varieties, including three-day, seven-day, and four-week versions. The organizers can have one or more slots per day. Most stroke survivors take medications once or twice a day; therefore, the most practical organizer would be a seven-day organizer with AM and PM slots. A stroke survivor should place his pill organizer in a spot where he does something every day. When he does this activity, seeing the pill box will remind him to take his medications. Pretty soon, taking them will become automatic.

Some pharmacies—even mail-order pharmacies—now prepare pills in little paper or plastic pockets with the date, day, and time of day that the medication should be taken. A pharmacist may also sell a device that will prompt a patient with a buzzer when he is due for medication. Of course, smart phones can be programmed to remind their owners of important events throughout the day.

A stroke survivor should never think, "Well, if I miss a dose no big deal. Or if I run out of a prescription, maybe I don't need it anymore. I don't feel any different without it." Remember, there are no immediate symptoms to alert someone of high blood pressure, high blood sugar, or improper blood clotting. If a patient misses a dose, he should ask his healthcare provider what to do. Some medications can be taken as soon as a patient remembers he missed a dose, others cannot. Sometimes a missed dose must simply remain missed, with a patient resuming his normal medication schedule upon his next dose.

A WARNING

A stroke patient should never stop a medication without checking with his healthcare provider first. Medications for high blood pressure, high blood sugar, or to keep his blood from clotting (including baby aspirin, if it has been prescribed by his healthcare provider) need to be taken at regular intervals. If he misses too many doses, he could have another stroke.

A patient or his loved one should establish a relationship with his healthcare provider's office staff or nurse so that he or his loved one can always call her with a question. She will either know the answer or will ask the healthcare provider and get back to him. So, if a patient thinks he is having an adverse reaction to one of his meds, he should let his healthcare provider know. It's possible his symptoms have nothing to do with his medications or, if they are related, his healthcare provider may change his prescription. Many healthcare systems have electronic patient portals through which a patient can ask his healthcare provider questions. If this option is available, a stroke survivor should not hesitate to take advantage of it.

Keeping All Therapy Visits

For stroke survivors, continuing therapies (OT, PT, ST) on an outpatient basis can mean the difference between making a lot of progress and losing any gains made before going home. Therapy is essential for him to get back as much of his old life as possible.

If a patient will not be seeing the same therapists from the hospital or rehabilitation center, his healthcare provider and former therapists may be able to recommend which centers would be best for him. A patient should get to know his new therapists enough that he feels comfortable asking them questions and doing what they recommend. If they give him work to do at home, he should feel confident that he is being steered in the right direction. If he really dislikes his therapist, he can ask to be assigned to a different one.

If a healthcare provider orders therapy, it will be covered by Medicare or private health insurance, which will continue to pay as long as a patient is making progress. This is one reason therapists give periodic tests to compare with previous tests. A patient can ask to see the results of these tests, which he may find rewarding and encouraging.

In some cases, therapists will be able to come to his home. Online exercise videos may also be helpful. For instance, if he is struggling with keyboarding, there are online sites that present passages to type, which are then scored to measure typing ability. A patient's first efforts may look jumbled, but results will improve with effort and a good sense of humor.

On non-therapy and non-doctor days, a patient could plan a trip to the hairdresser or barber. Nothing improves a person's morale more than a nice haircut. If his place of worship is important to him, he could find a way to get to services or ask for a visit from a religious leader.

Meeting Nutritional Needs

When a patient returns home, it is important for him to have access to nutritious food. If a loved one is not available to help and he cannot prepare meals for himself, a program such as *Meals on Wheels* may be an option. This volunteer-run service is offered to seniors in many communities across the country. Healthy, delicious homemade foods are delivered to a person's home once a day, with volunteers helping to put the food away in his refrigerator or cupboards, or on his counters where he can easily reach them. The cost will depend on his community and his ability to pay.

Most communities have restaurants that deliver, of course, and there are also third-party food delivery services that will pick up food at most restaurants that do not deliver. When ordering food, the focus should be on healthy meals. If a patient is able to cook at home but cannot get to the grocery store, many supermarkets can deliver groceries for a fee.

Arranging Transportation

If a patient cannot drive himself places, he will need to find someone who can take him to appointments and even out to lunch. This may be a spouse or a dear friend, or perhaps a neighbor. It may also be someone from his place of worship.

The community may offer special bus services for seniors, individuals with disabilities, or those who don't drive. They can pick him up at his home, help him enter the bus, take him to his appointment, and bring him home afterwards. There may or may not be a fee for usage of these buses. A hospital's social worker will be able to offer information on such services.

There are also taxis and rideshare services, but these can get costly. If the expense is manageable, these services can provide a patient with transportation to anywhere he needs to go, giving him independence. In some cases, they may even drive him to a different city to visit relatives or friends, and then bring him home.

DRIVING AFTER A TIA OR STROKE

Should someone who has experienced a TIA or stroke drive? It's important to check in with healthcare providers. Occupational therapists routinely assess whether their patients should drive. In fact, there are dedicated driving evaluations. Most states have laws that obligate healthcare providers to notify the Department of Public Health or the Department of Motor Vehicles if a patient has any deficits that would make driving difficult. Ultimately the Department of Motor Vehicles will make the determination whether or not to suspend a license. The following common problems associated with strokes can impair driving ability:

- Weakness

- Lack of sensation in a hand, arm, leg, or foot

- Vision difficulties, most commonly a visual field cut, where a stroke survivor doesn't see one half of the visual field

- Neglect (i.e., not paying attention to one side)

- Difficulty judging distances and how close objects are

- Slow reaction times

- Poor judgment

- Poor memory, poor concentration, confusion about road rules

- Inability to solve problems

- Fatigue that could interfere with responses

- Inability of the legs and feet to operate the gas and brake pedals quickly and correctly

- Inability of the arms and hands to steer carefully

- Inability to look from side to side quickly

- Changes to the sense of balance

A healthcare provider may require that a patient pass a driving test before she decides if he is ready to drive. She may want him to participate in therapy by an OT who is specially trained in helping people regain their driving skills. For example, the OT will likely have special gadgets to test the ability of a patient's feet to respond correctly to the gas and the brake pedals.

A therapist will also work on reaction time, which is the critical time between when you first see an object and when you respond. For example, the length of time between when a driver first sees a pedestrian and when he brakes is extremely important. Other matters that will be worked on include problem-solving, memory, and coordination. A patient's OT will keep in touch with his healthcare provider along the way, informing her of his progress so she can make a decision.

A stroke survivor should not drive if his healthcare provider has advised against doing so.

Getting Outside Help

A stroke survivor may have all kinds of help available to him in his everyday life. For example, if he is solely responsible for writing checks and keeping his check book balanced, his OT can provide special therapy in which he practices addition and subtraction from a practice checking account. A patient's spouse, family member, or trusted friend can also help him with this important chore until he can do it on his own.

Neighborhood teenagers can also help a stroke survivor with certain tasks, either for a fee or as community service. They can bring in newspapers and mail each day. They can take garbage out, rake leaves, or shovel snow. They can pick up groceries, feed pets, take dogs for walks, or clean litter boxes. They can mow lawns and weed gardens. They can even take stroke survivors on short neighborhood walks.

If a stroke survivor needs help getting dressed in the morning and getting his meals, he can hire someone to help him with his daily routine. He may need someone for only part of the day. He can also hire someone to do his house cleaning.

Using a Smart Speaker

A popular class of electronic devices is revolutionizing the way people obtain information, keep track of their chores and appointments, manage their home environments, and access entertainment. Referred to as "smart speakers," these devices are wireless speakers that respond to spoken commands by means of a virtual personal assistant.

Setting up a smart speaker requires a computer or mobile device of some sort. Once it has been set up, though, it can be used completely through voice commands and spoken questions, such as, "Set an alarm for 7 AM," "Play Gershwin's *Rhapsody in Blue*," "Set a reminder for me to take my pills at 9 AM and 6 PM," or, "What is the weather today in Eugene, Oregon?" Many of these services can be connected to smart home devices such as lights, thermostats, garage doors, sprinklers, or security systems.

Safeguarding Living Quarters

Technology has revolutionized the process of making a house or apartment more secure. By installing a front and back door camera, it is easy to see who is at the door without having to open the door. These devices also come in the form of a combined doorbell, camera, and speaker. When the doorbell rings, a smart phone or home computer can alert a stroke survivor to any visitors at his door and allow him to see and communicate with them, whether or not he is actually at home.

These monitoring devices are designed to be accessed by more than one person, so not only can a stroke survivor see who is at the door but so can his loved one—even though they may be living at a different location.

LIFTING MOOD AND REDUCING ISOLATION

Stroke survivors often have difficulties with mood and can feel isolated. Considering how different life can be after a stroke, these difficulties are more than understandable. It may take time to accept the stroke and establish a new normal. Adjustment isn't easy, but there are techniques that can help put patients in a good mindset.

Joining Support Groups

A stroke can leave a survivor feeling alone. Considering stroke estimates in the United States, however, which suggest that over 795,000 people experience a stroke each year and about 610,000 of these are first strokes, a survivor is anything but alone. Research has shown that people who participate in support groups or self-help programs generally handle things better than people who try to handle everything on their own. It is more than simply encouraging and supportive for a stroke survivor to interact with people who are facing similar challenges. Support groups can also offer valuable information. The people he meets may be able to tell him about good local healthcare providers, rehabilitation clinics, or coping strategies that work for them. He could share recipes for heart-healthy and brain-healthy foods, receive recipes from others, and develop new friendships. Often, stroke support groups invite experts in various fields to talk about topics of interest and answer questions. Online support groups are available as well.

Information on support groups for stroke survivors may be available at local hospitals or senior centers, or through healthcare providers. Of course, an online search should also yield helpful results.

Feeling Empowered

While a stroke refers to a medical event, it is also, in essence, a chronic condition, meaning its effects can last a long time. Many risk factors for stroke, including high blood pressure and type 2 diabetes, are also chronic conditions. One of the most helpful ways to manage a chronic condition is to feel like you have power over your own health. There are numerous "evidence-based programs" aimed at empowering individuals with chronic conditions. One example is the Chronic Disease Self-Management Program (CDSMP), an evidence-based self-management program originally developed at Stanford University. This program was created to help people with chronic conditions develop the skills and support to manage their own health. It's a six-week workshop in which people meet in a group for two and a half hours a week.

These workshops are facilitated by two peer leaders who either have chronic conditions themselves or have cared for someone with a chronic condition. Facilitators have all gone through rigorous training themselves to facilitate the workshops. During each workshop, techniques are taught for managing frustration, fatigue, pain, and isolation; talking with family, friends, and healthcare providers; managing medications; being physically active; eating a healthy diet; solving problems; and making decisions. Each person develops his own realistic short-term goals. In addition to empowering people to manage their own health, CDSMP workshops provide a support system of individuals facing similar challenges. CDSMP workshops are also helpful for caregivers. Workshops are offered across the United States. To find a workshop, consult the Self-Management Resource Center online at www.selfmanagementresource.com/programs/find-a-workshop.

Helping Others

Once a stroke survivor's symptoms—which can include problems with balance, strength, coordination, energy, and speech—have improved, he may feel the need to do something for others. Remember, as Saint Francis of Assisi said, "It is in giving that we receive," so if a stroke survivor can help others he, too, will also be helped. There are different ways to help, even if physical limitations are considerable. Time, life experience, and a caring ear are three things a stroke survivor can offer.

A house of worship or local community center can provide a list of "shut-ins" who would love to have a phone friend. Talking to someone who will listen can be a huge help to these individuals. They will be so glad to have a friend to converse with daily or weekly. As the Dalai Lama has said, "If you want others to be happy, practice compassion; if you want to be happy, practice compassion!"

For those who want to be helpful, there are many other ways of doing so. Examples include folding and stuffing envelopes for charities, lending artistic abilities to various non-profit publications, and being a part of a prayer chain to pray for those in distress.

Keeping the Faith

For many people, the role of faith holds an important place in their lives. Experiencing a stroke can certainly be a test of one's faith. To many, setting up connections to their religious roots can create a powerful source of hope, kinship, comfort, and acceptance. The power of belief is not without its miracles. It can overcome many things. Attending services can also encourage a stroke survivor to get involved in various activities sponsored by his place of worship.

Enjoying Reading, Music, and New Hobbies

A stroke survivor may enjoy watching TV, but we recommend he engage in other pastimes too. As far as TV goes, he should try to include shows that stretch his mind a little, like *Wheel of Fortune* or *Jeopardy*. He may enjoy informative shows on HGTV or National Geographic, or try comedy shows—after all, laughter is the best medicine. He should avoid shows that may depress him or elevate his blood pressure. In general, he should try not to sit in front of the TV for too long, no matter the programming.

If a patient likes to read, his friends could bring him books from the library or ones they have read. If the act of reading is more difficult, audiobooks may be the answer. Puzzles such as crosswords and Sudoku are also good pastimes, and many such puzzles can be found online. These types of activities are great for stimulating his brain and helping it to repair itself, and they fill the time in an enjoyable way.

Looking through old photo albums may help bring back memories of happy times with friends and family. If a stroke survivor has photos that need to be placed in albums, doing so would be a good hobby. If he is good with his hands, carving wood may be a satisfying hobby (but a therapist should be consulted first). Or he could learn to knit or crochet, which are very relaxing activities. Hooking rugs is another hobby that can be soothing. Patience is important when starting these hobbies, however, as hand coordination may make them difficult at first.

If a patient loves music, he should listen to whatever music makes him feel happy. If he can stand and chooses music with a strong rhythm, then he can sway to the beat. He could even dance if he is able. If he can only sit, he can clap his hands or keep time with his foot. If he plays an instrument, he could give it a try again. At first, it may be frustrating, as he may miss half the notes, but it's like anything—the more he practices, the better he will get as his abilities return. Rhythm also helps his brain to heal.

Other good pastimes include drawing, sketching, and painting. These hobbies don't have to produce great art but rather spur enjoyment in the mere act of creation. Writing fictional stories for children or adults, or perhaps a family history or recollections of a family trip, is a great idea, too. If typing is difficult at first, it will improve with practice.

If a stroke survivor was a golfer before his stroke, he could try some putting in his backyard. Being out in the fresh air will lift his mood. If he played tennis before his stroke, he could try to regain this ability. If tennis is just too much for him, perhaps pickleball would be a better fit. Pickleball is a little like badminton, ping pong, and tennis. A paddle and a ball are used, but the court is much smaller than a tennis court, making it easier to get around. His therapist should know if he has any sport-related goals, so she can use the right therapy to develop those skills again. Sporting activities require balance, coordination, and strength, which are good things to work on, whatever his future.

Some survivors even take up boxing, and some rehabilitation units have ways to hold a person upright in a harness so he can punch a bag, which can not only improve his balance and strength but also help him release some of his anger and frustration.

Advice for Caregivers
SEX AND INTIMACY

If you are the sexual partner of a stroke survivor, you may be wondering if his stroke will affect your sex life. Although you may be worried about the possibility, it is highly unlikely that having sex will cause another stroke. You may be worried you will somehow hurt him. You may be aware that he has had changes in his sensations and are wondering how these changes will affect your lovemaking. If depression is a problem for him, it may affect his sexual desires. Some medications will also reduce sexual desire and can cause impotence. Be sure to ask his healthcare provider if one of his medications could be causing this issue. It is important, so don't be embarrassed to have this discussion.

At first, your partner may not want to have actual intercourse but would rather cuddle or hug. If so, focus on hugging and cuddling, perhaps caressing and massaging him lovingly while telling him how much you love him. Laughter and playfulness can help if appropriate. Let things progress over time from there. You may need to alter positions to accommodate physical problems from the stroke. Enjoy experimentation and let him guide you.

Writing Down Three Good Things

Too often we dwell on unhappy things. Here is one easy way to improve a person's mood. It was devised by researchers at Duke University School of Medicine for their medical residents who were tired, stressed, and depressed. The members of one group of residents were told each to write down three good things that had happened that day before going to bed. A good thing might include the smile of a child, a pretty sunset, or a grateful patient. The group did this every night for a couple of months. When the researchers retested their moods and depression levels, the medical residents who had written down three good things every day showed a great deal of improvement compared with a group of residents who had not followed this routine. The researchers believed that by thinking of good things before bed, the medical residents would improve their sleep and be happier in the morning, and it seemed to do just that.

This technique could benefit a stroke survivor too, who may start to notice more and more good things throughout the day as a result of writing them down each night. As he looks for good things, he will also notice fewer things that disturb him.

The three good things don't have to be mind-blowing—being able to accomplish a goal in therapy, enjoying tasty berries, or enjoying a phone call are all good examples. And if writing is a problem, simply thinking of three good before drifting off to sleep can still be helpful.

INSURANCE, MEDICARE, AND MEDICAID

While they are the last thing a recovering stroke survivor should have to think about, medical bills are a stark reality that must be addressed. Having a stroke can be financially overwhelming. For survivors over sixty-five who have Medicare Part A (hospital insurance) and Part B (medical insurance), these plans should help cover many inpatient and outpatient costs, and even some at-home rehabilitation services. If a patient has additional health insurance coverage through an employer, he should contact the carrier to find out what it covers. If a stroke survivor is younger than sixty-five and does not have private insurance, he may qualify for Medicaid.

People who are at least sixty-five years old and receiving Social Security benefits are eligible for Medicare Part A, which covers hospital expenses such as a semi-private room, meals, nursing services, medications, and a number of other hospital services and supplies. Medicare Part A also covers limited home healthcare services such as part-time skilled nursing care; physical, speech, and occupational therapies; social services; part-time home health aide services, and medical equipment (paying 80 percent of the cost of equipment ordered by a doctor.) Under Part A, a doctor can order these home services only if a patient cannot leave his home.

Medicare Part B covers medical services and supplies such as outpatient care, ambulance services, and medical equipment. There is a monthly fee for Part B. To be eligible for Medicare Part B a person must be at least sixty-five years old and a US citizen or permanent resident who has been living continuously in the United States for the past five years.

If a stroke survivor cannot return to work, he may be eligible for Social Security Disability Insurance (SSDI) and Supplemental Security Income (SSI). Applications to these programs should be submitted as soon as possible after a stroke, as they may take three to five months to be processed. A patient must have been disabled for at least five full months before payments can begin. If he has received disability benefits from Social Security for at least twenty-four months in a row, he may be eligible for Medicare. If he receives Supplemental Security Income (SSI), he is eligible for Medicaid.

Advice for Caregivers
HELPING WITH FINANCES

Strokes are expensive—the average lifetime cost of an ischemic stroke has been estimated to be about $140,000. Your loved one will probably need you to help him work his way through the financial and insurance mazes. Just at a time when he doesn't need to have financial worries on top of his other concerns, he is expected to make major decisions that will affect his future and his family's future. Help him or find someone who can.

You can help him a lot by talking with his social worker, and perhaps making calls to Social Security and Medicare if needed. Help him fill out any necessary insurance forms. Be sure to help him keep all his bills and forms in one place—perhaps in a folder or envelope—so he can easily access them. Check them off after they have been paid. If his stroke has affected his ability to reason and think things through, he may need help writing checks and balancing his account. If he has a financial advisor, contact her, especially if tax time is near. Try to set up automatic bill payments online so that he doesn't need to write a check or remember to pay bills every month.

But what if a stroke survivor is many years younger than sixty-five and is now disabled? Such a patient may be eligible for Medicare if he has received disability benefits from Social Security or certain disability benefits from the Railroad Retirement Board (RRB) for at least twenty-four months in a row. He may also be eligible for Medicaid.

And what about prescriptions? Medicare A will cover the cost of medications while a patient is in the hospital or a skilled nursing facility. After he leaves, he may want to apply for Medicare Plan D, but this plan will not pay all prescription costs and has a monthly fee. Private insurance may also pay part of the cost of prescriptions. Finally, there is also the Prescription Assistance Program (PAP), which can help pay for prescription drugs if a person doesn't have health insurance or prescription drug coverage. These programs are offered by drug companies to provide free or low-cost drugs to patients who qualify.

FINDING SILVER LININGS

A stroke changes a survivor's life and the lives of those around him forever. Although it may sound strange to say, good things can come from a stroke. Ties between a married couple may be strengthened, as they will need each other more and in more profound ways. In addition, spouses who have depended so much upon their significant others to perform certain tasks, such as cooking, mowing the lawn, washing clothes, grocery shopping, may suddenly have to perform these tasks themselves. While it may be difficult to take on new responsibilities and accept changes in the roles each person plays in a couple, it could also lead to positive outcomes for both spouses, such as a greater appreciation of commitment and a fuller sense of self.

If a survivor has children or grandchildren, they will need to step up, too. Even young children can be helpful by bringing a recovering stroke patient something he needs, fixing him a healthy snack, or folding the laundry. Perhaps an older child can fix things around the house and take care of his car. If children live out of town, maybe they can help pay for some of the new expenses. All these methods of pitching in will bring a survivor's family closer together.

CONCLUSION

There are many ways for a stroke survivor to transition back to home and community life successfully and live well. A well-prepared home environment that is free of clutter can go a long way in ensuring a positive outcome in this situation. Establishing routines, staying organized, getting help, keeping in touch with family and friends, and strengthening a social network are all necessary parts of achieving a normal home life after a stroke. Nevertheless, it's important to remember that there may be unplanned setbacks—a fall, a missed appointment, a period of depression, etc.—but he can get past these moments if he simply accepts them, sees how far he has come, and continues to move forward.

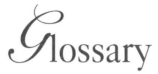Glossary

This book sometimes uses terms that are common in discussions of strokes but may not be completely familiar to you. You may hear these terms when discussing strokes with doctors or other healthcare professionals. To help you better understand strokes and their treatments, definitions are provided below for words that are often used by those who diagnose and treat strokes, and for words that are important in this book, all of which are noted by the use of *italic type* in the main text.

abdominal obesity. Excessive abdominal fat around the stomach and abdomen that can result in negative impacts to health.

ACE inhibitor. A medication that lowers blood pressure by preventing the formation of a hormone called *angiotensin II*.

acupoints. Specific points on the body that are targeted in *acupuncture* and *acupressure*.

acupressure. A complementary therapy in which fingertips rather than needles are used to stimulate *acupoints*.

acupuncture. A complementary therapy in which very fine stainless steel needles are placed at specific *acupuncture points*, or *acupoints*, to help the body heal.

acupuncture points. See *acupoints*.

advanced practice providers. The collective term used to describe *nurse practitioners* and *physician assistants*.

aerobic exercise. Exercise that increases the heart rate and increases oxygen intake, thereby benefiting the heart, brain, and muscles.

alteplase. A medication used for an *ischemic stroke.*

amyloid. A protein that can build up in the small *arteries* of the brain with age and lead to *intracerebral hemorrhages.*

aneurysm. An outpouching, or balloon-like bulge, of the wall of an *artery.*

angiotensin II. A hormone that is involved in numerous activities that increase blood pressure.

anterior cerebral artery. An *artery* that extends from the *internal carotid artery* and supplies blood to the frontal lobes of the brain.

anterior cerebral artery stroke. A stroke that is located in the territory of the *anterior cerebral artery.*

anticoagulant. A blood-thinning medication that slows the time it takes for blood to clot.

antioxidant. A substance that neutralizes a *free radical* by giving this unstable molecule an electron without becoming unstable itself.

antiplatelet. A blood-thinning medication that prevents *platelets* from clumping together.

antithrombotic. A medication that prevents *blood clots. Antiplatelet* and *anticoagulant* medications are collectively called antithrombotics.

aorta. The main *artery* originating from the heart.

aphasia. A condition characterized by difficulty understanding or formulating language.

arteries. Blood vessels that carry oxygen-rich blood to the body.

aspiration. A condition that occurs when liquid or food travels down the wrong pipe and enters the lungs rather than the stomach.

atherosclerosis. A condition in which hard plaques form in the arteries, causing the *arteries* to narrow over time.

atria. The two upper chambers of the heart.

atrial fibrillation. An abnormal heart rhythm in which the *atria* beat irregularly and often rapidly, allowing *blood clots* to form.

atrial flutter. An abnormal heart rhythm in which the *atria* beat rapidly and do not squeeze properly, allowing *blood clots* to form.

basilar artery. A single blood vessel that is formed by the union of the two *vertebral arteries* and feeds the *brainstem*.

behavioral therapy. A type of therapy that helps a person change bad habits, replacing them with healthy ones.

blood clot. A thick clump of blood that forms after an injury and "plugs" the hole at the injured site.

body mass index (BMI). A measure of a person's relative size based on weight and height.

brainstem. The posterior part of the brain that is continuous with the spinal cord. It allows signals to travel between the brain and the spinal cord.

calcium channel blocker. A medication that prevents calcium from entering the cells of the heart and blood vessel walls, thus relaxing the *arteries* and lowering blood pressure.

capillaries. The smallest blood vessels in the body, which carry nutrients and oxygen to tissues and remove waste products.

cardioembolic stroke. A stroke caused by a *blood clot* originating in the heart.

case manager. A healthcare team member who collaboratively assesses, plans, facilitates, and coordinates services to meet a patient's comprehensive health needs.

Circle of Willis. A formation of arteries located at the base of the brain, where the main arteries leading to the brain connect.

clergy. A group of people who have been ordained for religious duties.

cognitive behavioral therapy (CBT). A problem-focused and action- oriented type of therapy. It helps subjects develop skills to alter the way they think about and react to situations.

cognitive distortion. A belief, thought, or attitude that causes a person to perceive reality inaccurately.

complementary medicine. Nonstandard therapies that are meant to be used alongside traditional treatment options.

comprehensive stroke center. A stroke center that offers even more specialized services than those available at a *primary stroke center.*

computed tomography scan (CT scan). A type of x-ray scan that combines a series of x-ray images to provide detailed information on the bones, tissues, and fluid in the body.

constraint-induced movement therapy (CIMT). A type of therapy in which a patient's unaffected (or less affected) limb is put in a mitt or sling in order to encourage his affected limb to attempt particular movements.

contracture. A tightening or shortening of muscles, causing joint stiffness, and difficulty moving.

CT angiogram. A *CT scan* in which contrast dye is injected into a vein and scans are taken that show the contrast dye moving through the blood vessels, revealing areas of narrowing or occlusion.

deep vein thrombosis (DVT). A *blood clot* formed in a deep vein in the body (typically a vein in a leg).

direct oral anticoagulant. A type of blood-thinning medication that requires less monitoring than traditional blood thinners.

dissection. A tear in a blood vessel.

dysarthria. A condition characterized by slurred speech.

dysphagia. A condition characterized by difficulty swallowing.

edema. Fluid accumulation and swelling.

embolism. A blockage of a blood vessel, typically by a *blood clot.*

embolus. A piece of a *blood clot* that has broken off and can travel to a smaller blood vessel, eventually causing a blockage known as an embolism.

endocarditis. Inflammation of the heart valves.

excitatory signals. Signals sent by the brain and spinal cord to muscles that result in contraction of those muscles.

fine motor skills. The abilities of the small muscles in the fingers, hands, and wrists to do various activities

free radical. A molecule with an uneven number of electrons that can steal an electron from another molecule, causing it to become a free radical.

functional electrical stimulation (FES). The electrical stimulation of a weak or paralyzed muscle.

gait. A person's manner of walking.

glycemic index (GI). A ranking system of the carbohydrates found in different foods that is meant to help determine how a food will affect blood glucose levels.

glycemic load (GL). A ranking system that reflects not only the *glycemic* index of a food but also the amount of carbohydrates contained in a designated portion of food, providing a measurement that includes both the quality and quantity of a food's carbohydrates.

heart attack. A blockage that deprives the heart of oxygen.

heart failure. A condition in which the heart works less efficiently than normal.

hemoglobin A1c. A blood test that determines a person's average blood sugar level over the past three months.

hemorrhagic stroke. A stroke caused by a weakened blood vessel that has burst, causing bleeding in the brain.

high blood pressure. A condition in which the long-term force of blood against artery walls is high enough to lead to health problems such as stroke.

high-density lipoprotein (HDL) cholesterol. A type of cholesterol that carries cholesterol from other parts of the body back to the liver, which then removes this cholesterol from the body. It is often referred to as "good" cholesterol.

homocysteine. An amino acid that can increase stroke risk by making the blood more prone to clotting and accelerating *atherosclerosis.*

hyperbaric oxygen therapy (HBOT). A type of therapy in which a patient is exposed to 100 percent oxygen in a whole-body chamber under extra atmospheric pressure.

hypertension. See *high blood pressure.*

hypertriglyceridemia. A condition characterized by high *triglycerides* in the blood.

infective endocarditis. *Endocarditis* caused by an infection in the blood.

inhibitory signals. Signals sent by the brain and spinal cord to muscles that result in the relaxation of those muscles.

intensive care unit (ICU). A specialized section of a hospital that provides comprehensive and continuous care for persons who are critically ill.

intermittent pneumatic compression. A device used to prevent *blood clots* in deep veins.

internal carotid artery. A paired *artery* (one on each side of the head) that is located at the front, or anterior, of the brain.

intracerebral hemorrhage. A *hemorrhagic stroke* that bleeds into the brain.

intrauterine device. A contraceptive device.

ischemic stroke. A stroke caused by a blockage of an *artery* leading to the brain, depriving the brain of oxygen.

large artery atherosclerosis. Plaque build-up in the walls of *arteries* leading to the brain.

large vessel stroke. A stroke caused by a blockage of one of the main arteries leading to the brain.

left atrial ablation. A procedure that is meant to treat the symptoms of *atrial fibrillation.*

left atrial appendage. An outpouching of the left atrium, or top left chamber of the heart.

left middle cerebral artery stroke. A stroke caused by a blockage of the left middle cerebral *artery*, often leading to weakness and numbness on the right side, *aphasia*, and difficulty seeing the right visual field.

left occipital lobe. The left side of the occipital lobe. It is responsible for vision in the right visual field.

left sensory cortex. The sensory cortex of the left hemisphere. It receives and interprets information from the right side of the body.

licensed practical nurse (LPN). A nurse who has completed a state-approved training program, which results in either a diploma, certificate, or associate's degree. Known as a *licensed vocational nurse* in some states.

licensed vocational nurse (LVN). A nurse who has completed a state-approved training program, which results in either a diploma, certificate, or associate's degree. Known as a *licensed practical nurse* in some states.

living will. A document that allows an individual to communicate his healthcare wishes in the event that he is unable to do so due to illness.

low-density lipoprotein (LDL) cholesterol. A type of cholesterol that can lead to a build-up of plaque in *arteries.*

magnetic resonance imaging (MRI). A medical imaging technique that uses strong magnetic fields and radio waves to produce three-dimensional pictures of the inside of the body.

medical assistant. An individual who works with a healthcare team and has been trained to take vital signs, administer basic care, and report any concerns to *registered nurses* and physicians.

mental imagery. Imagining doing tasks without doing them.

metabolic syndrome. A group of health conditions that commonly occur together (high blood pressure, abdominal obesity, abnormal cholesterol, and high blood sugar) and increase a person's risk of heart disease, stroke, and type 2 diabetes.

middle cerebral artery. A paired *artery* (one on each side of the head) that branches out from the *internal carotid artery.* It is one of the three major paired *arteries* that supply blood to the brain.

motivational interviewing. A type of therapy that gets a subject to examine how he feels about any changes he is hoping to make. By asking pointed questions, a therapist can elicit a patient's uncertainties and hesitancies, which may stop him from making these changes.

music therapy. A type of therapy in which music is used to treat patients who have motor, speech, cognitive, or mood problems.

myelinated fibers. Cell parts that work like electrical wires transmitting signals.

nasal cannula. An oxygen-delivery device that consists of a small plastic tube that splits into two prongs, which are placed in the nostrils.

neglect. Problems processing sensory information that comes from one side of the body.

neurons. The fundamental building blocks of the nervous system. Also called nerve cells or brain cells, neurons specialize in the transmission of information throughout the body.

neuropathy. Damage to the nerves.

neuroplasticity. A property of the brain that allows it to form new networks throughout life.

neuroprotectant. A substance that protects brain cells.

nicotine replacement therapy (NRT). A type of therapy that provides alternative ways to deliver low doses of nicotine, keeping cravings under control and allowing a smoker to refrain from smoking.

nurse practitioner. A nurse who is licensed to do many of the tasks physicians do, such as treating patients independently and prescribing medication.

obese. Excessively overweight, which is defined as having a BMI of $30 \text{ kg}/\text{m}^2$ or greater.

occlusion. A blockage of a blood vessel.

occupational therapist (OT). A therapist who focuses on a stroke survivor's motor, cognitive, and psychological impairments that limit his ability to engage in activities, including social participation.

overweight. Exceeding a healthy body weight, which is defined as having a BMI between 25 and $29.9 \text{ kg}/\text{m}^2$.

oxidative stress. A condition characterized by high levels of *free radicals*, which can cause substantial damage to cells.

paradoxical embolism. An *embolism*, or blockage of a blood vessel, which occurs when a *blood clot* in the veins of the legs or pelvis travels through the heart or lungs to the brain.

paroxysmal atrial fibrillation. Intermittent *atrial fibrillation.*

patent foramen ovale (PFO). A connection between the left and right *atria.*

perfusion. The passage of fluid through the circulatory system to an organ or tissue.

person-centered therapy. A type of therapy in which a therapist relates to her client without hiding behind a professional façade; offers acceptance to a patient without expressing disapproval, judgment, or advice; and expresses empathy. It encourages a patient to feel comfortable enough to express himself without fear of judgment.

physical therapist (PT). A therapist who generally helps with walking and balance, and often provide exercises for strength and range of motion of affected limbs.

physician assistant. A healthcare provider who is licensed to treat patients and prescribe medication, but who may do so only in collaboration with a supervising physician.

placebo. A medically inactive substance or procedure that may nevertheless result in a benefit psychologically.

plasma. A yellow liquid that makes up approximately 55 percent of blood and carries nutrients such as glucose, proteins, fatty acids, and so on.

plaque. A substance made up of fat, cholesterol, calcium, and other materials in the blood, which begins to accumulate in the *arteries* with age, hardening and narrowing them.

platelets. A component of blood that helps prevent excessive bleeding after an injury.

pneumonia. An infection of the lungs.

posterior cerebral artery. A paired *artery* (one found on each side of the head) that is located at the back, or posterior, of the brain, arising from the *basilar artery*.

posterior cerebral artery stroke. A stroke caused by a blockage of a *posterior cerebral artery*, causing difficulty with vision and memory.

power of attorney. A legal document that allows an individual to appoint someone else as manager of his affairs, provided he is considered legally capable of making this decision.

prediabetes. A condition that is a precursor to type 2 diabetes.

primary stroke center. A certified hospital-based center with the resources to care for acute stroke patients.

reaction time. The length of time between first seeing or hearing an object and reacting to it.

recombinant tissue plasminogen activator (rtPA). A *tissue plasminogen* *activator* that is manufactured in a laboratory. It is a key treatment for patients with ischemic stroke in the first four and half hours after symptom onset.

red blood cell. A component of blood that gives it its color and is responsible for carrying oxygen to all cells.

registered dietitian (RD). A healthcare provider who is trained in the science of nutrition and has studied at length the specific nutritional needs of someone who has special medical needs.

registered nurse (RN). A nurse who has obtained a nursing degree after finishing a two-year associate's degree program in nursing or a four-year bachelor's degree program in nursing.

rehabilitation. The process in which stroke survivors work on restoring their bodies and brains so that they can either return to their former lives or develop new, meaningful, and fulfilling new lives.

reversible vasoconstriction syndrome. A syndrome characterized by a sudden narrowing of the *arteries* of the brain, causing strokes.

right middle cerebral artery stroke. A stroke caused by a blockage of the right middle cerebral *artery*, resulting in weakness and numbness on the left side, neglect, and difficulty seeing the left visual field.

right motor cortex. The motor cortex of the right hemisphere. It is the area of the brain principally involved in the planning and execution of voluntary movement of the left side of the body.

right occipital lobe. The right side of the occipital lobe. It is responsible for vision in the left visual field.

selective serotonin reuptake inhibitor (SSRI). A type of medication that is used to treat depression.

small vessel disease. Narrowing of the small *arteries* that originate from the larger *arteries* leading to the brain.

social worker. An expert who is trained to help a patient, his family, and his caregivers find resources and services, and navigate the healthcare system. She is also licensed to provide counseling.

spasticity. An abnormal increase in muscle tone or stiffness of a muscle.

speech-language pathologist (SLP). See *speech therapist.*

speech therapist (ST). A therapist who addresses three main areas: swallowing, speech, and cognition (the ability to think and process information).

statin. A type of medication typically prescribed to lower cholesterol in the blood.

stent retriever. An expandable wire-mesh tube used in the mechanical removal of a *blood clot.*

subarachnoid hemorrhage. A *hemorrhagic stroke* that bleeds into the space between the brain and the skull.

subcutaneously. Under the skin.

subluxation. A partial dislocation.

supportive therapy. A type of therapy that simply reinforces a patient's healthy and adaptive patterns of thought.

synapses. The connections between nerve cells, or *neurons.*

systemic lupus erythematosus. A rheumatologic condition that can cause *endocarditis.*

thiazide diuretic. A blood pressure medication that directly affects the kidneys, lowering their ability to reabsorb sodium and chloride (the compound of which is known as salt), which the kidneys release into the urine.

thrombectomy. The removal of a *blood clot* via mechanical device.

thrombectomy-capable center. A stroke center that has been certified to perform a procedure known as *mechanical thrombectomy,* or pulling a *blood clot* out of a blood vessel.

thrombolytic. A type of medication that can dissolve *blood clots.*

thrombus. A thick clump of blood that forms after an injury and "plugs" the hole at the injured site, commonly known as a *blood clot.*

tissue plasminogen activator (tPA). An enzyme the body produces to help dissolve *blood clots.*

transcranial direct current stimulation. Stimulation of the brain through the use of electrical currents.

transcranial magnetic stimulation (TMS). Stimulation of the brain through the use of magnetic pulses.

transesophageal echocardiogram. A type of ultrasound that is done under sedation and involves putting a camera down the throat to look at the heart.

transient ischemic attack (TIA). A temporary disruption in blood flow to the brain, resulting in stroke symptoms that do not persist.

triglycerides. A type of fat in the blood that is stored in fat cells and released for energy production between meals.

type 2 diabetes. A condition in which the body does not use the hormone insulin properly, leading to consistently high blood sugar levels.

urinary tract infection. An infection of any part of the urinary system.

vasospasm. A condition in which arterial spasm results in constriction of the affected *arteries.*

vertebral artery. A paired *artery* (one found on each side) located in the neck. The two *vertebral arteries* join to form the *basilar artery,* which supplies the *brainstem.*

water pill. See *thiazide diuretic.*

white blood cell. A component of blood that helps the body fight infections.

white coat hypertension. A condition in which a patient's blood pressure reading is elevated in a doctor's office but returns to normal levels outside a healthcare setting.

Resources

A number of organizations and websites provide a wealth of information about stroke, its risk factors, its management, and other topics of interest to a stroke patient and his caregivers. This section provides a list of these resources. It includes resources that will help a stroke survivor meet his nutritional needs through food and supplements, break unhealthy habits, connect with a support group, and learn about exercises and other techniques that can aid in recovery. When it comes to strokes, knowledge truly is power.

GENERAL STROKE INFORMATION

American Heart Association

Website: www.heart.org

The purpose of the American Heart Association is to help reduce disability and death from cardiovascular diseases, including stroke.

American Stroke Association

Website: www.stroke.org

The American Stroke Association, a division of the American Heart Association, is focused on reducing disability and death from stroke.

Brain & Life: Neurology for Everyday Living

Website: www.brainandlife.org

This free magazine published by the American Academy of Neurology provides information about balance, exercise, and motivation, and relates inspiring personal stories for stroke patients and patients with other neurological disorders, and offers specific help and advice for their caregivers. Just click on "The Magazine" to read the current issue and browse past issues.

Caregiver Guide to Stroke

Website: www.stroke.org/we-can-help/caregivers-and-family/careliving-guide

This publication by the American Stroke Association is available online for free and a valuable source of information for recovering stroke patients and their caregivers.

Harvard Medical School Reports

Website: www.health.harvard.edu/special-health-reports

Harvard Medical School publishes easy-to-follow reports on a wide range of topics of interest for stroke patients. They are available for purchase at the above-referenced web address.

CAREGIVERS AND CARE FACILITIES

A Place for Mom

Website: www.aplaceformom.com

A Place for Mom is a free senior care referral service based in Seattle. It has information about more than 17,000 senior housing and eldercare providers throughout the United States and Canada.

Visiting Angels

Website: www.visitingangels.com

Visiting Angels is a national organization that helps seniors stay in their homes. They offer help in the home for a few hours a day or 24/7, and provide assistance with patient care, getting simple meals, taking clients for short walks, helping with home exercises, and doing light housework or errands.

STROKE SUPPORT GROUPS

American Heart Association— Support Network

Website: https://supportnetwork. heart.org

This free social network sponsored by the American Heart Association allows stroke survivors to read about other survivors' stories and share their own stories if they so choose.

American Stroke Association— Stroke Support Group Finder

Website: www.stroke.org/en/ stroke-support-group-finder

Stroke survivors can use this section of the American Stroke Association's website to search for stroke support groups by entering a zip code and a mile radius to narrow down the search area.

THERAPY ANIMALS

Alliance of Therapy Dogs

Website: www.therapydogs.com

This organization offers testing, certification, registration, support, and insurance to members who volunteer with their dogs in animal-assisted activities. It provides therapy dog services at no cost to facilities that need them.

Pet Partners

Website: https://petpartners.org

Pet Partners is the largest nonprofit registering therapy dogs and other therapy animal pets, including horses, cats, rabbits, and birds. Pet Partners trains volunteers and evaluates them with their pets for visiting animal programs in hospitals, nursing homes, veterans' centers, hospice, Alzheimer's facilities, courtrooms, schools and other settings.

SETTING UP GOOGLE ALERTS

Google—Alerts

Website: www.google.com/alerts

Using Google Alerts is a great way to learn about new stroke research and receive breaking information about the treatment of stroke and its risk factors. By entering specific search terms, you can direct Google to email you articles, blogs, videos, etc., pertaining to those subjects when they appear online.

BALANCE EXERCISES

Flint Rehab

Website: www.flintrehab.com/2018/
regaining-balance-after-stroke

Flint Rehab's "Recovery Blog" discusses causes of imbalance after stroke, how to cope with imbalance, and exercises that can improve imbalance.

BRAIN EXERCISES

Children's Storybooks Online

Website: www.magickeys.com/books

A survivor who is struggling with reading can try these delightful children's books free online. Reading aloud can be very helpful.

Free Web Arcade

Website: www.freewebarcade.com

Free Web Arcade is a gaming website that can help improve a survivor's abilities to think and react quickly. For example, the game "Sheep Dash" can help improve reaction time. Immediate scoring allows the player to keep track of how he may be improving. There are also games available that can help with language ability, including "Scrabble" and "Wheel of Fortune."

Math is Fun

Website: www.mathsisfun.com

This website is designed for those who are struggling with math. The user can choose different grade levels to match their abilities. This website also offers many puzzles and games.

RED LIGHT - GREEN LIGHT
Reaction Time Test

Website: https://faculty.washington.edu/chudler/java/redgreen.html

This free online game measures reaction time to a changing traffic light and keeps track of scores to mark improvement over time. The website also has other brain games, including jigsaw puzzles, card games, Monopoly, etc.

Typing.com

Website: www.typing.com/student/lessons

If a survivor's ability to type has been affected by a stroke, this website can help. It offers simple typing lessons and typing games. There are also tests designed to see how a person is improving.

Typing Test

Website: www.keyhero.com/free-typing-test

This website measures typing ability and gives practice sheets to help improve keyboarding performance.

EYE EXERCISES

College of Optometrists in Vision Development

Website: www.covd.org

This website helps users locate vision therapists in their areas.

Flint Rehab

Website: www.flintrehab.com/2019/eye-exercises-after-stroke

Flint Rehab's "Recovery Blog" offers numerous articles on stroke recovery, including those on eye exercises.

Neuro-Optometric Vision Rehabilitation

Website: https://nora.memberclicks.net/find-a-provider#

This website helps users locate nearby optometrists who are trained in vision therapy after a stroke.

Tactus Therapy—Visual Attention Therapy

Website: https://tactustherapy.com/app/vat

This app helps patients retrain their brains with interactive cancellation exercises that assess and treat left neglect.

Vision Tap

Website: http://www.visiontap.net/

Vision Tap is an app made up of a collection of vision-related procedures and may be used as part of a vision therapy program.

wikiHow—How to Rehab Vision Post Stroke

Website: www.wikihow.com/Rehab-Vision-Post-Stroke#Doing_Exercises_to_Improve_Vision_sub

This website suggests free exercises that can improve vision problems. It also discusses various types of vision therapy available from professionals.

PHYSICAL EXERCISES

American Physical Therapy Association

Website: http://aptaapps.apta.org/findapt/SearchResults.aspx

This website uses a survivor's zip code or city and state to help locate a local physical therapist.

Donna Brooks: Yoga for Stroke Recovery

Website: www.youtube.com/watch?v=DjpOmpXzI2A

Donna Brooks demonstrates how yoga can improve movement in a stroke patient.

Flint Rehab

Website: www.flintrehab.com/2020/stroke-exercises

Flint Rehab's "Recovery Blog" offers numerous articles on stroke recovery, including those on physical exercises. It also provides free downloadable stroke rehab exercises. The entire blog is a wealth of information.

Stroke Class

Website: www.strokeclass.com

This website provides at-home exercises for stroke patients as demonstrated by a physical therapist. It also offers videos on other stroke-related subjects.

Tai Chi Productions

Website: https://us.taichiproductions.com/dvds

This website sells online streaming video Tai Chi lessons with expert Dr. Paul Lam to aid in recovery from ill health, including stroke.

Wayne, Peter, with Mark L. Feurst. *The Harvard Medical School Guide to Tai Chi.* Boulder, CO: Shambhala, 2013.

This book offers a basic tai chi program illustrated by photographs, advice on how to integrate tai chi into daily life, summaries of research on the benefits of tai chi, and more.

Wei, Marilyn, and James E. Groves. *The Harvard Medical School Guide to Yoga.* Boston: Da Capo Lifelong Books, 2017.

This guide to yoga offers a science-based eight-week program designed to increase flexibility, enhance muscle and bone strength, improve sleep, enrich brain health, and aid in stress management. It includes illustrations of yoga sequences and principles of yoga safety.

PAIN RELIEF

Central Post-Stroke Pain Syndrome

Website: www.uspharmacist.com/ article/central- poststroke-pain-syndrome

Written by a pharmacist, this website discusses different drugs that may help post-stroke pain. It also discusses non-drug therapies.

Stroke Foundation—Pain after Stroke Fact Sheet

Website: https://strokefoundation. org.au/en/About-Stroke/Help-after-stroke/My-Stroke-Journey-fact-sheets/ Pain-after-stroke-fact-sheet

This resource discusses types of pain that can occur after a stroke and lists various pain treatment options.

BEHAVIORAL THERAPIES

Alcoholics Anonymous

Website: www.aa.org

The aim of this international organization is to help people get sober and stay sober. Its website features a search option to help people find AA groups in their particular locations.

American Lung Association

Website: www.lung.org/stop-smoking

This section of the American Lung Association's website contains advice and support from people who have had years of experience helping smokers quit. It also offers a telephone hotline for questions about lung health and help finding local healthcare.

Centers for Disease Control and Prevention

Website: www.cdc.gov/tobacco/ quit_smoking/index.htm

This section of the CDC's website offers information on how to quit smoking, tips on quitting from former smokers, advice on how to manage cravings after quitting, and a telephone number to call for support in quitting.

MyFinessPal

Website: www.myfitnesspal.com

This website offers helpful tools to lose weight and keep it off, such as a calorie counter and diet tracker. Membership is free and includes a mobile app, which allows users to log meals and exercise on the go.

National Heart, Lung, and Blood Institute

Website: www.nhlbi.nih.gov/health-pro/guidelines/current/obesity-guidelines/e_textbook/txgd/4323.htm

The NHLBI provides an overview of the behavioral therapy strategies used in weight loss and weight maintenance programs.

PsychCentral—5 Cognitive Behavioral Strategies for Losing Weight That Work

Website: https://psychcentral.com/blog/5-cognitive-behavioral-strategies-for-losing-weight-that-work

This resource provides information on how to approach and manage the process of losing weight.

Substance Abuse and Mental Health Services Administration (SAMHSA)

Website: www.samhsa.gov/find-help/national-helpline

The purpose of SAMHSA is to provide information on substance use or mental disorders and where to find treatment services for these issues. Its national helpline offers free, confidential treatment referrals.

MEDITATION

Insight Timer

Website: https://insighttimer.com

This app provides free access to a vast library if guided meditations to help with sleep problems, anxiety, and stress.

Smiling Mind

Website: www.smilingmind.com.au

Smiling Mind is a 100% non-for-profit organization that offers a free meditation app developed by psychologists and educators to help both children and adults reduce their stress levels and improve their well-being through mindfulness meditation.

UCLA Health—UCLA Mindful App

Website: www.uclahealth.org/marc/ucla-mindful-app

This easy-to-use app allows users to practice mindfulness meditation anywhere, anytime with the guidance of the UCLA Mindful Awareness Research Center.

NUTRITION, SUPPLEMENTS, AND RECIPES

American Heart Association Diet and Lifestyle Recommendations

Website: www.heart.org/en/healthy-living/healthy-eating/eat-smart/nutrition-basics/aha-diet-and-lifestyle-recommendations

This resource explains how a healthy diet and lifestyle are the best weapons to fight cardiovascular disease.

ConsumerLab.com

Website: www.consumerlab.com

Compiled by an organization independent of supplement manufacturers, ConsumerLab.com offers up-to-date research reports on various nutrients, including vitamins, minerals, and herbs. The website also compares many products by brand. An annual subscription fee is required for full access.

EatingWell

Website: www.EatingWell.com

Through its website, the publisher of EatingWell magazine offers healthy recipes that can be easily adapted to suit the AHA diet.

Harvard T.H. Chan School of Public Health—The Nutrition Source

Website: www.hsph.harvard.edu/ nutritionsource

This resource offers breaking nutrition news, articles on relevant subjects such as sodium and fiber, tips for maintaining a healthy weight, and recipes that can be adapted to the AHA diet.

National Heart, Lung, and Blood Institute

Website: https://healthyeating. nhlbi.nih.gov

The "Delicious Heart Health Recipes" section of this website provides wholesome recipes, including some from a variety of ethnic cuisines.

WebMD—Food Calculator

Website: www.webmd.com/diet/ healthtool-food-calorie-counter

This calculator quickly provides the calorie, fat, carbohydrate, and protein contents for over 37,000 foods and beverages.

AUDIOBOOKS

Audible

Website: www.audible.com

Audible sells digital audiobooks, radio and TV programs, and audio versions of magazines and newspapers.

The National Library Service for the Blind and Print Disabled

Website: www.loc.gov/nls

This amazing service offers hundreds of thousands of braille and talking books for free. These books may be downloaded to a smart phone or other listening device, or mailed at no cost.

Penguin Random House

Website: www.penguinrandomhouse.com/books/audiobooks

The Penguin Random House website features a wide variety of audiobooks available for purchase.

DRIVING

Driving after Stroke Stroke Association United Kingdom

Website: www.stroke.org.uk/sites/ default/files/driving_after_stroke.pdf

This website answers many questions about driving safely a stroke.

Senior Driving AAA

Website: https://seniordriving.aaa.com

The purpose of this website by AAA is to help seniors drive safer and longer. Seniors and their families will find lots of helpful information about challenges seniors face while driving.

$\mathscr{R}$eferences

Chapter 1

Giles MF, Rothwell PM. "Risk of stroke early after transient ischaemic attack: a systematic review and meta-analysis." *Lancet Neurol.* 2007 Dec;6(12):1063–1072.

O'Donnell MJ, Xavier D, Liu L, et al. "Risk factors for ischaemic and intracerebral haemorrhagic stroke in 22 countries (the INTERSTROKE study): a case-control study." *Lancet* Jul 10 2010;376(9735):112–123.

Saver JL. "Time is Brain-Quantified." *Stroke* 2006;37:263–266.

Virani SS, Alonso A, Benjamin EJ, et al. "Heart Disease and Stroke Statistics-2020 Update: A Report From the American Heart Association." *Circulation* 2020 Mar 3;141(9):e139–e596.

Wu CM, McLaughlin K, Lorenzetti DL, Hill MD, Manns BJ, Ghali WA. "Early risk of stroke after transient ischemic attack: a systematic review and meta-analysis." *Arch Intern Med* 2007 Dec 10;167(22):2417–2422.

Chapter 2

Billinger SA, Arena R, Bernhardt J, et al. "Physical activity and exercise recommendations for stroke survivors: a statement for healthcare professionals from the American Heart Association/American Stroke Association." *Stroke* 2014 Aug;45(8):2532–2553.

Brainin M, et al. "Multi-level community interventions for primary stroke prevention: A conceptual approach by the World Stroke Organization." *International Journal of Stroke* 2019 Sep 9.14(8):818–825.

Bushnell C, McCullough LD, Awad IA, et al. "Guidelines for the prevention of stroke in women: a statement for healthcare professionals from the American Heart Association/American Stroke Association." *Stroke* 2014 May;45(5):1545–1588.

Emdin CA, Rahimi K, Neal B, Callender T, Perkovic V, Patel A. "Blood pressure lowering in type 2 diabetes: a systematic review and meta-analysis." *JAMA* 2015 Feb 10;313(6):603–615.

Feigin VL, Krishnamurthi R, Bhattacharjee R, et al. "New Strategy to Reduce the Global Burden of Stroke." *Stroke* 2015;46:1740–1747.

Guo Y, Yue XJ, Li HH, et al. "Overweight and Obesity in Young Adulthood and the Risk of Stroke: a Meta-analysis." *J Stroke Cerebrovasc Dis* 2016 Dec;25(12):2995–3004.

Khoury JC, Kleindorfer D, Alwell K, et al. "Diabetes mellitus: a risk factor for ischemic stroke in a large biracial population." *Stroke* 2013 Jun;44(6):1500–4.

Kulshreshtha A, et al. "Family History of Stroke and Cardiovascular Health in a National Cohort." *J Stroke Cerebrovasc Dis* 2015 Feb;24(2):447–54.

Lin AM, Lin MP, Markovic D, et al. "Less than Ideal: Trends in Cardiovascular Health Among US Stroke Survivors." *Stroke* 2019;50:5–12.

Lin MP, Ovbiagele B, Markovic D, Towfighi A. "Association of Secondhand Smoke with Stroke Outcomes." *Stroke* 2016 Nov;47(11):2828–2835.

Lloyd-Jones DM, Hong Y, Labarthe D, et al. "Defining and setting national goals for cardiovascular health promotion and disease reduction: the American Heart Association's strategic Impact Goal through 2020 and beyond." *Circulation* 2010;121:586–613.

Marso SP, Kennedy KF, House JA, McGuire DK. "The effect of intensive glucose control on all-cause and cardiovascular mortality, myocardial infarction and stroke in persons with type 2 diabetes mellitus: a systematic review and meta-analysis." *Diab Vasc Dis Res* 2010 Apr;7(2):119–130.

Meschia JF, Bushnell C, Boden-Albala B, et al. "Guidelines for the primary prevention of stroke: a statement for healthcare professionals from the American Heart Association/American Stroke Association." *Stroke* 2014 Dec;45(12):3754–3832.

O'Donnell MJ, Chin SL, Rangarajan S, et al. "Global and regional effects of potentially modifiable risk factors associated with acute stroke in 32 countries (INTERSTROKE): a case-control study." *Lancet* 2016 Aug 20;388(10046):761–775.

Oxley TJ, Mocco J, Majidi, S, et al. "Large-vessel Stroke as a Presenting Feature of Covid-19 in the Young." *NEJM* epub April 28, 2020.

Rashid P, Leonardi-Bee J, Bath P. "Blood pressure reduction and secondary prevention of stroke and other vascular events: a systematic review." *Stroke* 2003 Nov;34(11):2741–8.

Spitzer RL, Kroenke K, Williams JB. "Validation and utility of a self-report version of PRIME-MD: the PHQ primary care study. Primary Care Evaluation of Mental Disorders. Patient Health Questionnaire." *JAMA* 1999 Nov 10;282(18):1737–44.

Towfighi A, Ovbiagele B, et al. "Poststroke Depression: A Scientific Statement for Healthcare Professionals from the American Heart Association/American Stroke Association." *Stroke* 2017 Feb;48(2): e30–e43.

Virani SS, Alonso A, Benjamin EJ, et al. "Heart Disease and Stroke Statistics-2020 Update: A Report From the American Heart Association." *Circulation* 2020 Mar 3;141(9):e139–e596.

Whelton PK, Carey RM, Aronow WS, et al. "2017 ACC/AHA/AAPA/ABC/ACPM/AGS/APhA/ASH/ASPC/NMA/PCNA Guideline for the Prevention, Detection, Evaluation, and Management of High Blood Pressure in Adults: A Report of the American College of Cardiology/American Heart Association Task Force on Clinical Practice Guidelines." *Hypertension* 2018 Jun;71(6):1269–1324.

Chapter 3

Hemphill JC, Greenberg SM, Anderson, C, et al. "Guidelines for the Management of Spontaneous Intracerebral Hemorrhage: A Guideline for Healthcare Professionals From the American Heart Association/American Stroke Association." *Stroke* 2015;46:2032–2060.

Kernan WN, Ovbiagele B, Black HR, et al. "Guidelines for the prevention of stroke in patients with stroke and transient ischemic attack: a guideline for healthcare professionals from the American Heart Association/American Stroke Association." *Stroke* 2014;45:2160–2236.

Powers WJ, et al. "Guidelines for the Early Management of Patients With Acute Ischemic Stroke: 2019 Update to the 2018 Guidelines for the Early Management of Acute Ischemic Stroke: A Guideline for Healthcare Professionals From the American Heart Association/American Stroke Association." *Stroke* 2019 Dec;50(12):e440–e441.

Powers WJ, Rabinstein AA, Ackerson T, et al. "2018 Guidelines for the Early Management of Patients With Acute Ischemic Stroke: A Guideline for Healthcare Professionals From the American Heart Association/American Stroke Association." *Stroke* 2018;49:246–e110.

Chapter 4

Winstein CJ, Stein J, Arena R, et al. "Guidelines for Adult Stroke Rehabilitation and Recovery: A Guideline for Healthcare Professionals From the American Heart Association/American Stroke Association." *Stroke* 2016 Jun;47(6):e98–e169.

Chapter 5

Winstein CJ, Stein J, Arena R, et al. "Guidelines for Adult Stroke Rehabilitation and Recovery: A Guideline for Healthcare Professionals From the American Heart Association/American Stroke Association." *Stroke* 2016 Jun;47(6):e98–e169.

Chapter 6

Winstein CJ, Stein J, Arena R, et al. "Guidelines for Adult Stroke Rehabilitation and Recovery: A Guideline for Healthcare Professionals From the American Heart Association/American Stroke Association." *Stroke* 2016 Jun;47(6):e98–e169.

Chapter 7

Brady MC, et al. "Speech and language therapy for aphasia after stroke." *Cochrane Database Syst Rev* 2016 Jun 1;(6):CD000425.

Das Nair R, et al. "Cognitive rehabilitation for memory deficits after stroke." *Cochrane Database Syst Rev* 2016 Sep; 2016(9): CD002293.

Nasreddine ZS, Phillips NA, Bédirian V, et al. "The Montreal Cognitive Assessment, MoCA: a brief screening tool for mild cognitive impairment." *J Am Geriatr Soc* 2005 Apr;53(4):695–9.

Pendlebury ST, et al. "Methodological Factors in Determining Risk of Dementia After Transient Ischemic Attack and Stroke: (II) Effect of Attrition on Follow-Up." *Stroke* 2015 Jun;46(6):1494–500.

Pendlebury ST, Rothwell PM. "Prevalence, incidence, and factors associated with pre-stroke and post-stroke dementia: a systematic review and meta-analysis." *Lancet Neurol* 2009 Nov;8(11):1006–18.

Tombaugh TN, McDowell I, Kristjansson B, et al. "Mini-Mental State Examination

(MMSE) and the Modified MMSE (3MS): A psychometric comparison and normative data." *Psychological Assessment* 1996;8(1):48–59.

Winstein CJ, Stein J, Arena R, et al. "Guidelines for Adult Stroke Rehabilitation and Recovery: A Guideline for Healthcare Professionals From the American Heart Association/American Stroke Association." *Stroke* 2016 Jun;47(6):e98–e169.

Chapter 8

Biller J, Sacco RL, Albuquerque FC, et al. Cervical arterial dissections and association with cervical manipulative therapy: a statement for healthcare professionals from the American Heart Association/American Stroke Association." *Stroke* 2014 Oct;45(10):3155–3174.

Fotakopoulos G, Kotlia P. "The Value of Exercise Rehabilitation Program Accompanied by Experiential Music for Recovery of Cognitive and Motor Skills in Stroke Patients." *J Stroke Cerebrovasc Dis* 2018 Nov;27(11):2932–2939.

Kasper S, Gastpar M, Muller WE, et al. "Lavender oil preparation Silexan is effective in generalized anxiety disorder—a randomized, double-blind comparison to placebo and paroxetine." *Int J Neuropsychopharmacol* 2014 Jun;17(6):859–869.

Love MF, et al. "Mind-body interventions, psychological stressors, and quality of life in stroke survivors: a systematic review." *Stroke* 2019 Feb;50(2):434–440.

Magee WL, Clark I, Tamplin J, Bradt J. "Music interventions for acquired brain injury." *Cochrane Database Syst Rev* 2017 Jan 20;1:CD006787.

Sibbritt D, Peng W, Lauce R, Ferguson C, Frawley J, Adams J. "Efficacy of acupuncture for lifestyle risk factors for stroke: A systematic review." *PLoS One* 2018 Oct 26;13(10):e0206288.

Taylor-Piliae RE, Hoke TM, Hepworth JT, Latt LD, Najafi B, Coull BM. "Effect of Tai Chi on physical function, fall rates and quality of life among older stroke survivors." *Arch Phys Med Rehabil* 2014 May;95:816–824.

Woelk H, Schlafke S. "A multi-center, double-blind, randomised study of the Lavender oil preparation Silexan in comparison to Lorazepam for generalized anxiety disorder." Phytomedicine 2010 Feb;17(2) 94–9.

Yang A, Wu HM, Tang JL, Xu L, Yang M, Liu GJ. "Acupuncture for stroke rehabilitation." *Cochrane Database Syst Rev* 2016 Aug 26;(8):CD004131.

Chapter 9

Amarenco P, Bogousslavsky J, Callahan A 3rd, et al. "Stroke Prevention by Aggressive Reduction in Cholesterol Levels (SPARCL) Investigators. High-dose atorvastatin after stroke or transient ischemic attack." *N Engl J Med* 2006 Aug 10;355(6):549–59.

Antithrombotic Trialists' Collaboration. "Collaborative meta-analysis of randomised trials of antiplatelet therapy for prevention of death, myocardial infarction, and stroke in high risk patients." *BMJ* 2002 Jan 12;324(7329):71–86.

Antithrombotic Trialists' (ATT) Collaboration, Baigent C, Blackwell L, et al. "Aspirin in the primary and secondary prevention of vascular disease: collaborative meta-analysis of individual participant data from randomised trials." *Lancet* 2009 May 30;373(9678):1849–1860.

Chollet F, Tardy J, Albucher JF, et al. "Fluoxetine for motor recovery after acute ischaemic stroke (FLAME): a randomised placebo-controlled trial." *Lancet Neurol* 2011 Feb;10:123–30. Erratum in: *Lancet Neurol* 2011 Mar;10(3):205.

FOCUS Trial Collaboration. "Effects of fluoxetine on functional outcomes after acute stroke (FOCUS): a pragmatic, double-blind, randomised, controlled trial." *Lancet* 2019 Jan 19;393(10168):265–274.

Fox CS, Golden SH, Anderson C, et al. Update on Prevention of Cardiovascular Disease in Adults With Type 2 Diabetes Mellitus in Light of Recent Evidence: A Scientific Statement From the American Heart Association and the American Diabetes Association. *Diabetes Care* 2015 Sep;38(9):1777–803.

Goyal M, Singh S, Sibinga EM, et al. "Meditation programs for psychological stress and well-being: a systematic review and meta-analysis." *JAMA Intern Med* 2014 Mar;174(3):357–368.

Hopper I, Billah B, Skiba M, Krum H. "Prevention of diabetes and reduction in major cardiovascular events in studies of subjects with prediabetes: meta-analysis of randomised controlled clinical trials." *Eur J Cardiovasc Prev Rehabil.* 2011 Dec;18(6):813–823.

Kelley GA, Kelley KS. "Exercise and sleep: a systematic review of previous meta-analyses." *J Evid Based Med* 2017 Feb;10(1):26–36.

Kernan WN, Ovbiagele B, Black HR, et al. "Guidelines for the prevention of stroke in patients with stroke and transient ischemic attack: a guideline for healthcare professionals from the American Heart Association/American Stroke Association." *Stroke* 2014 Jul;45(7):2160–2236.

Kernan WN, Viscoli CM, Furie KL, et al. "Pioglitazone after Ischemic Stroke or Transient Ischemic Attack." *N Engl J Med* 2016 Apr 7;374(14):1321–1331.

Li Y, Pan A, Wang DD, et al. "Impact of Healthy Lifestyle Factors on Life Expectancies in the US Population." *Circulation* 2018 Jul 24;138(4):345–355.

Lin MP, Ovbiagele B, Markovic D, Towfighi A. "Life's Simple 7" and Long-Term Mortality After Stroke." *J Am Heart Assoc* 2015;4(11).

Moresoli P, Habib B, Reynier P, Secrest MH, Eisenberg MJ, Filion KB. "Carotid Stenting Versus Endarterectomy for Asymptomatic Carotid Artery Stenosis: A Systematic Review and Meta-Analysis." *Stroke* 2017 Aug;48(8):2150–2157.

Rothwell PM, Eliasziw M, Gutnikov SA, et al. "Analysis of pooled data from the randomised controlled trials of endarterectomy for symptomatic carotid stenosis." *Lancet* 2003 Jan 11;361(9352):107–116.

Seer P, Raeburn JM. "Meditation training and essential hypertension: a methodological study." *J Behav Med* 1980 Mar;3(1):59–71.

Siebenhofer A, Jeitler K, Horvath K, et al. "Long-term effects of weight-reducing drugs in people with hypertension." *Cochrane Database Syst Rev* 2016 Mar 2;3:CD007654.

Sinha SS, Jain AK, Tyagi S, Gupta SK, Mahajan AS. "Effect of 6 Months of Meditation on Blood Sugar, Glycosylated Hemoglobin, and Insulin Levels in Patients of Coronary Artery Disease." *Int J Yoga* 2018 May–Aug;11(2):122–128.

Towfighi A, Ovbiagele B, et al. "Poststroke Depression: A Scientific Statement for Healthcare Professionals from the American Heart Association/American Stroke Association." *Stroke* 2017 Feb;48(2):e30–e43.

Ventegodt S, Merrick J. "Lifestyle, quality of life, and health." *ScientificWorldJournal* 2003;3:811–825.

Whelton PK, et al. "2017 ACC/AHA/AAPA/ABC/ACPM/AGS/APhA/ASH/ASPC/NMA/PCNA Guideline for the Prevention, Detection, Evaluation, and Management of High Blood Pressure in Adults: Executive Summary: A Report of the American College of Cardiology/American Heart Association Task Force on Clinical Practice Guidelines." *Hypertension* 2018 Jun;71(6):1269–1324.

Wilk AI, Jensen NM, Havighurst TC. "Meta-analysis of randomized control trials addressing brief interventions in heavy alcohol drinkers." *J Gen Intern Med* 1997 May;12(5):274–283.

Chapter 10

Adriouch S, Lampure A, Nechba A, et al. "Prospective Association between Total and Specific Dietary Polyphenol Intakes and Cardiovascular Disease Risk in the Nutrinet-Sante French Cohort." *Nutrients* 2018 Oct 29;10(11).

American Diabetes Association. "Standards of Medical Care in Diabetes—2019." *Diabetes Care* 2019 Jan; 42 (Suppl. 1).

Chen GC, Lu DB, Pang Z, Liu QF. "Vitamin C intake, circulating vitamin C and risk of stroke: a meta-analysis of prospective studies." *J Am Heart Assoc* 2013 Nov 27;2(6):e000329.

Choe H, Hwang JY, Yun JA, et al. "Intake of antioxidants and B vitamins is inversely associated with ischemic stroke and cerebral atherosclerosis." *Nutr Res Pract* 2016 Oct;10(5):516–523.

Costello RB, Dwyer JT, Bailey RL. "Chromium supplements for glycemic control in type 2 diabetes: limited evidence of effectiveness." *Nutr Rev* 2016 Jul;74(7):455–68.

Han B, Lyu Y, Sun H, Wei Y, He J. "Low serum levels of vitamin D are associated with post-stroke depression." *Eur J Neurol* 2015 Sep;22(9):1269–1274.

Hankey GJ, Eikelboom JW, Baker RI, et al. "B vitamins in patients with recent transient ischaemic attack or stroke in the VITAmins TO Prevent Stroke (VITATOPS) trial: a randomised, double-blind, parallel, placebo-controlled trial." *Lancet Neurol* 2010;9(9): 855–865.

Hertog MG, Feskens EJ, Hollman PC, Katan MB, Kromhout D. "Dietary antioxidant flavonoids and risk of coronary heart disease: the Zutphen Elderly Study." *Lancet* 1993 Oct 23;342(8878):1007–1011.

Hooper L, et al. "Omega-6 fats for the primary and secondary prevention of cardiovascular disease." *Cochrane Database of Syst Rev* 2018 Jul 18; 7:CD011094.

Hooper L, Kay C, Abdelhamid A, et al. "Effects of chocolate, cocoa, and flavan-3-ols on cardiovascular health: a systematic review and meta-analysis of randomized trials." *Am J Clin Nutr* 2012 Mar;95(3):740–751.

Hou LQ, Liu YH, Zhang YY. "Garlic intake lowers fasting blood glucose: meta-analysis of randomized controlled trials." *Asia Pac J Clin Nutr* 2015;24(4):575–582.

Hsu CY, Chiu SW, Hong KS, et al. "Folic Acid in Stroke Prevention in Countries without Mandatory Folic Acid Food Fortification: A Meta-Analysis of Randomized Controlled Trials." *J Stroke* 2018;20(1):99–109.

Jenkins DJA, Spence JD, Giovannucci EL, et al. "Supplemental Vitamins and Minerals for CVD Prevention and Treatment." *J Am Coll Cardiol* 2018 Jun 5;71(22):2570–2584.

Jorat MV, Tabrizi R, Mirhosseini N, et al. "The effects of coenzyme Q10 supplementation on lipid profiles among patients with coronary artery disease: a systematic review and meta-analysis of randomized controlled trials." *Lipids Health Dis* 2018 Oct 9;17(1):230.

Kimble R, Keane KM, Lodge JK, Howatson G. "Dietary intake of anthocyanins and risk of cardiovascular disease: A systematic review and meta-analysis of prospective cohort studies." *Crit Rev Food Sci Nutr* 2019;59(18):3032–3043.

Larsson SC, Virtamo J, Wolk A. "Chocolate consumption and risk of stroke: a prospective cohort of men and meta-analysis." *Neurology* 2012 Sep 18;79(12):1223–1229.

Leppala JM, Virtamo J, Fogelholm R, et al. "Controlled trial of alpha-tocopherol and beta-carotene supplements on stroke incidence and mortality in male smokers." *Arterioscler Thromb Vasc Biol* 2000 Jan;20(1):230–235.

Leppala JM, Virtamo J, Fogelholm R, et al. "Vitamin E and beta carotene supplementation in high risk for stroke: a subgroup analysis of the Alpha-Tocopherol, Beta-Carotene Cancer Prevention Study." *Arch Neurol* 2000 Oct;57(10):1503–1509.

Makariou SE, Michel P, Tzoufi MS, Challa A, Milionis HJ. "Vitamin D and stroke: promise for prevention and better outcome." *Curr Vasc Pharmacol* 2014 Jan;12(1):117–124.

Mozaffarian D. "Dietary and policy priorities for cardiovascular disease, diabetes, and obesity: a comprehensive review." *Circulation* 2016 Jan 12;133:187–225.

Navas-Acien A, Bleys J, Guallar E. "Selenium intake and cardiovascular risk: what is new?" *Curr Opin Lipidol* 2008 Feb;19(1):43–49.

Newberry SJ. "What is the evidence that vitamin C supplements lower blood pressure?" *Am J Clin Nutr* 2012 May;95(5):997–998.

Ohira T, Peacock JM, Iso H, Chambless LE, Rosamond WD, Folsom AR. "Serum and dietary magnesium and risk of ischemic stroke: the Atherosclerosis Risk in Communities Study." *Am J Epidemiol* 2009 Jun 15;169(12):1437–1444.

Ovbiagele B, Starkman S, Teal P, et al. "Serum calcium as prognosticator in ischemic stroke." *Stroke* 2008 Aug;39(8):2231–2236.

Park JH, Saposnik G, Ovbiagele B, et al. "Effect of B-vitamins on stroke risk among individuals with vascular disease who are not on antiplatelets: A meta-analysis." *Int J Stroke* 2016;11(2):206–211.

Park KY, Chung PW, Kim YB, et al. "Serum Vitamin D Status as a Predictor of Prognosis in Patients with Acute Ischemic Stroke." *Cerebrovasc Dis* 2015;40(1-2):73–80.

Poole KE, Loveridge N, Barker PJ, et al. "Reduced vitamin D in acute stroke." *Stroke* 2006 Jan;37(1):243–245.

Ren Y, et al. "Chocolate consumption and risk of cardiovascular diseases: a meta-analysis of prospective studies." *Heart* 2019 Jan;105:49–55.

Reiter RJ, Tan DX, Galano A. "Melatonin: exceeding expectations." *Physiology (Bethesda)* 2014 Sep;29(5):325–333.

Ried K, Sullivan TR, Fakler P, Frank OR, Stocks NP. "Effect of cocoa on blood pressure." *Cochrane Database Syst Rev* 2012 Aug 15;(8):CD008893.

Ried K, Toben C, Fakler P. "Effect of garlic on serum lipids: an updated meta-analysis." *Nutr Rev* 2013 May;71(5):282–299.

Rosique-Esteban N, Guasch-Ferre M, Hernandez-Alonso P, Salas-Salvado J. "Dietary Magnesium and Cardiovascular Disease: A Review with Emphasis in Epidemiological Studies." *Nutrients* 2018 Feb 1;10(2).

Saber H, Yakoob MY, Shi P, et al. "Omega-3 Fatty Acids and Incident Ischemic Stroke and Its Atherothrombotic and Cardioembolic Subtypes in 3 US Cohorts." *Stroke* 2017 Aug;48:2678–2685.

Serban MC, Sahebkar A, Zanchetti A, et al. "Effects of Quercetin on Blood Pressure: A Systematic Review and Meta-Analysis of Randomized Controlled Trials." *J Am Heart Assoc* 2016 Jul 12;5(7):pii: e002713.

Singh S, Arora RR, Singh M, Khosla S. "Eicosapentaenoic Acid Versus Docosahexaenoic Acid as Options for Vascular Risk Prevention: A Fish Story." *Am J Ther* 2016 May–Jun;23(3):e905–910.

Sluijs I, Czernichow S, Beulens JW, et al. "Intakes of potassium, magnesium, and calcium and risk of stroke." *Stroke* 2014 Feb;45(4):1148–1150.

Spence JD, Yi Q, Hankey GJ. "B vitamins in stroke prevention: time to reconsider." *Lancet Neurol* 2017 Sep;16(9):750–760.

Suksomboon N, Poolsup N, Yuwanakorn A. "Systematic review and meta-analysis of the efficacy and safety of chromium supplementation in diabetes." *J Clin Pharm Ther* 2014 Jun;39(3):292–306.

Sun Q, Pan A, Hu FB, Manson JE, Rexrode KM. "25-Hydroxyvitamin D levels and the risk of stroke: a prospective study and meta-analysis." *Stroke* 2012 Jun;43(6):1470–1477.

Toole JF, Malinow MR, Chambless LE, et al. "Lowering homocysteine in patients with ischemic stroke to prevent recurrent stroke, myocardial infarction, and death: the Vitamin Intervention for Stroke Prevention (VISP) randomized controlled trial." *JAMA* 2004; 291(5):565–575.

Willett WC. "The role of dietary n-6 fatty acids in the prevention of cardiovascular disease." *J Cardiovasc Med (Hagerstown)* 2007 Sep;8 Suppl 1:S42–45.

Xiao Y, et al. "Circulating Multiple Metals and Incident Stroke in Chinese Adults." *Stroke* 2019 Jul;50(7):1661–1668.

Xiong XJ, Wang PQ, Li SJ, Li XK, Zhang YQ, Wang J. "Garlic for hypertension: A systematic review and meta-analysis of randomized controlled trials." *Phytomedicine* 2015 Mar 15;22(3):352–361.

Yue W, Xiang L, Zhang YJ, Ji Y, Li X. "Association of serum 25-hydroxyvitamin D with symptoms of depression after 6 months in stroke patients." *Neurochem Res* 2014 Nov;39(11):2218–2224.

Zeng R, Xu CH, Xu YN, Wang YL, Wang M. "The effect of folate fortification on folic acid-based homocysteine-lowering intervention and stroke risk: a meta-analysis." *Public Health Nutr* 2015 Jun;18(8):1514–1521.

Zhao M, Wu G, Li Y, et al. Meta-analysis of folic acid efficacy trials in stroke prevention: Insight into effect modifiers." *Neurology* 2017;88(19):1830–1838.

Chapter 11

Bernstein AM, de Koning L, Flint AJ, Rexrode KM, Willett WC. "Soda consumption and the risk of stroke in men and women." *Am J Clin Nutr* 2012 May;95(5):1190–1199.

Bernstein AM, Pan A, Rexrode KM, et al. "Dietary protein sources and the risk of stroke in men and women." *Stroke* 2012 Mar;43(3):637–644.

Borgeraas H, Johnson LK, Skattebu J, Hertel JK, Hjelmesaeth J. "Effects of probiotics on body weight, body mass index, fat mass and fat percentage in subjects with overweight or obesity: a systematic review and meta-analysis of randomized controlled trials." *Obes Rev* 2018 Feb;19(2): 219–32.

Ericson U, Hellstrand S, Brunkwall L, Schulz CA, Sonestedt E, Wallstrom P, Gullberg B, Wirfalt E, Orho-Melander M. "Food sources of fat may clarify the inconsistent role of dietary fat intake for incidence of type 2 diabetes." *Am J Clin Nutr* 2015 May;101(5):1065–80.

Estruch R, et al. "Primary Prevention of Cardiovascular Disease with a Mediterranean Diet Supplemented with Extra-Virgin Olive Oil or Nuts." *N Engl J Med* 2018 Jun 21;378(25):e34.

Geng T, Qi L, Huang T. "Effects of dairy products consumption on body weight and body composition among adults: an updated meta- analysis of 37 randomized controlled trials." *Mol Nutr Food Res* 2018:62(1).

Johnson RK, Appel LJ, Brands M, et al. "Dietary sugars intake and cardiovascular health: a scientific statement from the American Heart Association." *Circulation* 2009 Sep 15;120(11):1011–1020.

Johnson RK , Lichtenstein AH , et al. "Low-Calorie Sweetened Beverages and Cardiometabolic Health: A Science Advisory from the American Heart Association." *Circulation* 2018 Aug 28;138(9):e126–e140.

Nettleton JA, Brouwer IA, Geleijnse JM, Hornstra G. "Saturated Fat Consumption and Risk of Coronary Heart Disease and Ischemic Stroke: A Science Update." *Ann Nutr Metab* 2017;70(1):26–33.

Mozaffarian D. "Dairy Foods, Obesity, and Metabolic Health: The Role of the Food Matrix Compared with Single Nutrients." *Adv Nutr* 2019 Sep 1;10(5):917S–923S.

Pase MP, Himali JJ, Beiser AS, et al. "Sugar- and Artificially Sweetened Beverages and the Risks of Incident Stroke and Dementia: A Prospective Cohort Study." *Stroke* 2017 May;48(5):1139–1146.

Te Morenga LA, Howatson AJ, Jones RM, Mann J. "Dietary sugars and cardiometabolic risk: systematic review and meta-analyses of randomized controlled trials of the effects on blood pressure and lipids." *Am J Clin Nutr* 2014 Jul;100(1):65–79.

Van Horn L, Carson JS, Appel LJ, et al. "Recommended Dietary Pattern to Achieve Adherence to the American Heart Association/American College of Cardiology (AHA/ACC) Guidelines A Scientific Statement From the American Heart Association." *Circulation* 2016;134:e505–e529.

Chapter 12

Afshin A, Micha R, Khatibzadeh S, Mozaffarian D. "Consumption of nuts and legumes and risk of incident ischemic heart disease, stroke, and diabetes: a systematic review and meta-analysis." *Am J Clin Nutr* 2014 Jul;100(1):278–288.

Al-Waili N, Salom K, Al-Ghamdi A, Ansari MJ, Al-Waili A, Al-Waili T. "Honey and cardiovascular risk factors, in normal individuals and in patients with diabetes mellitus or dyslipidemia." *J Med Food* 2013 Dec;16(12):1063–1078.

Estruch R, et al. "Primary Prevention of Cardiovascular Disease with a Mediterranean Diet Supplemented with Extra-Virgin Olive Oil or Nuts." *N Engl J Med* 2018;378(25):e34.

Kokubo Y, Iso H, Saito I, et al. "The impact of green tea and coffee consumption on the reduced risk of stroke incidence in Japanese population: the Japan public health center-based study cohort." *Stroke* 2013;44:1369–1374.

Larsson SC. "Coffee, Tea, and Cocoa and Risk of Stroke." *Stroke* 2014;45:309–314.

Mozaffarian D. "Dairy Foods, Obesity, and Metabolic Health: The Role of the Food-Matrix Compared with Single Nutrients." *Adv Nutr* 2019 Sep 1;10(5):917S–923S.

Van Horn L, Carson JS, Appel LJ, et al. "Recommended Dietary Pattern to Achieve Adherence to the American Heart Association/American College of Cardiology (AHA/ACC) Guidelines A Scientific Statement From the American Heart Association." *Circulation* 2016;134:e505–e529.

Chapter 14

Allida S, Cox KL, Hsieh CF, Lang H, House A, Hackett ML. "Pharmacological, psychological, and non-invasive brain stimulation interventions for treating depression after stroke." *Cochrane Database of Systematic Reviews* 2020, Issue 1. Art. No.: CD003437.

Almeida OP, Marsh K, Alfonso H, Flicker L, Davis TM, Hankey GJ. "B-vitamins reduce the long-term risk of depression after stroke: The VITATOPS-DEP trial." *Ann Neurol* 2010 Oct;68(4):503–510.

Chollet F, Tardy J, et al. "Fluoxetine for motor recovery after acute ischaemic stroke (FLAME): a randomised placebo-controlled trial." *Lancet Neurol* 2011 Feb;10(2):123–130.

Gooneratne NS. "Complementary and alternative medicine for sleep disturbances in older adults." *Clin Geriatr Med* 2008 Feb;24(1):121–138, viii.

Gu Y, Zhao K, Luan X, et al. "Association between Serum Magnesium Levels and Depression in Stroke Patients." *Aging Dis* 2016 Dec;7(6):687–690.

Han B, Lyu Y, Sun H, Wei Y, He J. "Low serum levels of vitamin D are associated with post-stroke depression." *Eur J Neurol* 2015 Sep;22(9):1269–1274.

Harrison RA, Field TS. "Post stroke pain: identification, assessment, and therapy." *Cerebrovasc Dis* 2015;39(3-4):190–201.

Katzman MA, et al. "Canadian clinical practice guidelines for the management of anxiety, posttraumatic stress and obsessive-compulsive disorders." *BMC Psychiatry* 2014, 14(Suppl 1):S1.

Li Y, Lv MR, Wei YJ, et al. "Dietary patterns and depression risk: A meta-analysis." *Psychiatry Res* 2017 Jul;253:373–382.

Markisic M, Pavlovic AM, Pavlovic DM. "The Impact of Homocysteine, Vitamin B12, and Vitamin D Levels on Functional Outcome after First-Ever Ischaemic Stroke." *Biomed Res Int* 2017;2017:5489057.

Nii M, Maeda K, Wakabayashi H, Nishioka S, Tanaka A. "Nutritional Improvement and Energy Intake Are Associated with Functional Recovery in Patients after Cerebrovascular Disorders." *J Stroke Cerebrovasc Dis* 2016 Jan;25(1):57–62.

Rajizadeh A, Mozaffari-Khosravi H, Yassini-Ardakani M, Dehghani A. "Effect of magnesium supplementation on depression status in depressed patients with magnesium deficiency: A randomized, double-blind, placebo-controlled trial." *Nutrition* 2017 Mar;35:56–60.

Towfighi A, Ovbiagele B, et al. "Poststroke Depression: A Scientific Statement for Healthcare Professionals from the American Heart Association/American Stroke Association." *Stroke* 2017 Feb;48(2): e30–e43.

Yue W, Xiang L, Zhang YJ, Ji Y, Li X. "Association of serum 25-hydroxyvitamin D with symptoms of depression after 6 months in stroke patients." *Neurochem Res* 2014 Nov;39(11):2218–2224.

Chapter 15

Hill VA, Towfighi A. "Modifiable Risk Factors for Stroke and Strategies for Stroke Prevention." *Semin Neurol* 2017 Jun;37(3):237–258.

Lorig K, Sobel DS, et al. "Evidence suggesting that a chronic disease self-management program can improve health status while reducing hospitalization: a randomized trial." *Med Care* 1999 Jan;37(1):5–14.

Towfighi A, Cheng EM, et al. "Randomized controlled trial of a coordinated care intervention to improve risk factor control after stroke or transient ischemic attack in the safety net: Secondary stroke prevention by Uniting Community and Chronic care model teams Early to End Disparities (SUCCEED)." *BMC Neurol* 2017 Feb 6;17(1):24.

Towfighi A. "Stroke Prevention." *Semin Neurol* 2017 Jun;37(3):235–236.

About the Authors

Amytis Towfighi, MD, received her bachelor's degree from MIT and her MD from Johns Hopkins School of Medicine. She completed internship in Internal Medicine at Massachusetts General Hospital, neurology residency at Massachusetts General Hospital and Brigham and Women's Hospital, and vascular neurology fellowship at UCLA. She is currently an associate professor of neurology and the James and Dorothy Williams Stroke Scholar at the Keck School of Medicine of the University of Southern California. Dr. Towfighi is director of neurological services for the Los Angeles County Department of Health Services, and associate medical director of research, associate medical director of neurological services, and chief of neurology at Los Angeles County+USC Medical Center. She served as chair of neurology at Rancho Los Amigos National Rehabilitation Center for eleven years. While Dr. Towfighi's research focuses on stroke prevention, she is also committed to empowering stroke survivors and transforming healthcare systems to provide seamless patient-centered care.

Laura J. Stevens, MSci, received her master's degree in nutrition science from Purdue University. She has worked at Purdue as a researcher, investigating the relationship between diet and health disorders. Apart from her work at Purdue, Laura is the author of eight books on diet, behavior, and allergies. She lives with her amazing cat, Bentley, in Lafayette, Indiana.

Index

recombinant tissue plasminogen activator (rtPA), 45–46
red blood cell, 7, 46
red meat, 188–189
registered dietitian (RD), 66, 144, 180
registered nurse (RN), 63–64
rehabilitation, 54–70, 72–73, 80–83, 89, 92–97, 102, 109, 111, 119–121, 146, 180, 190, 209, 250–251, 255–256, 258, 263, 266, 268
reversible vasoconstriction syndrome, 136
right middle cerebral artery stroke, 12–13
right motor cortex, 11
right occipital lobe, 11
risk factors, 18–20, 30, 33, 35, 37–38, 52, 120, 126–152, 163, 170, 175, 199, 208, 213, 264
  managing, with behavioral therapy, 141–147
  managing, with food, 149–150
  managing, with lifestyle tips, 151–152
  managing, with medication, 126–136
  managing, with meditation, 148–149
  managing, with physical therapy, 136–141
  managing, with supplements, 150–151

salt. *See* sodium.
selective serotonin reuptake inhibitor (SSRI), 130, 239, 242
sex, after stroke, 266
sleep, after stroke, 244–248
small vessel disease, 9
smoking, 22–24, 33, 44, 120, 126, 132, 134–136, 140–142, 144–145, 147, 242
social worker, 65–66, 72, 112, 142, 144, 235, 260, 269
sodium, 19, 179–182
spasticity, 60–61, 93, 235, 242, 244
speech-language pathologist (SLP). *See* speech therapist.

speech therapy (ST), 42, 62, 65, 68, 72–73, 97–113, 119, 258
statin, 53–54, 109, 123, 128, 169
stent retriever, 46
stroke center. *See* comprehensive stroke center; primary stroke center.
subarachnoid hemorrhage, 10, 48–49
subcutaneous, 42, 50
subluxation, 61, 235, 243
sugar, 182–188
supportive care, 41, 49
supportive therapy, 143
swallowing, after stroke, 97–99
synapses, 15, 55
systemic lupus erythematosus, 36

thiazide diuretic, 132–133
thrombectomy, 15, 44, 46
thrombectomy-capable center, 15
thrombolytic, 44–45
thrombus, 7
tissue plasminogen activator (tPA), 45
transcranial direct current stimulation, 58–59
transcranial magnetic stimulation (TMS), 58–59
transesophageal echocardiogram, 53
transient ischemic attack (TIA), 10, 17, 21, 31, 38, 126, 131, 133, 136–137, 260
triglycerides, 25–27, 53, 128, 165–166, 168, 199, 208, 212–213
type 2 diabetes. *See* diabetes, type 2.

urinary tract infection, 49–50, 246

vasospasm, 48–49
vertebral artery, 120
vision, after stroke, 11–14, 79, 260
vitamins, protective, 153–160

water pill. *See* thiazide diuretic.
white blood cell, 7
white coat hypertension, 22

Other Square One Titles of Interest

What You Must Know About Vitamins, Minerals, Herbs and So Much More

SECOND EDITION

Choosing the Nutrients That Are Right for You

Pamela Wartian Smith, MD, MPH

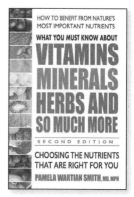

Even if you follow a healthful diet, you are probably not getting all the nutrients you need to prevent disease. Why? There are many reasons, ranging from the mineral-depleted soils in which our foods are grown, to medications that rob the body of various vitamins and minerals. Reflecting the latest scientific research, *What You Must Know About Vitamins, Minerals, Herbs and So Much More—Second Edition* explains how you can restore and maintain health through the wise use of nutrients. Whether you are trying to overcome a medical condition or you simply want to preserve good health, this book will guide you in making the best dietary and supplement choices.

$16.95 US • 512 pages • 6 x 9-inch paperback • ISBN 978-0-7570-0471-1

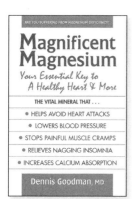

Magnificent Magnesium

Your Essential Key to a Healthy Heart & More

Dennis Goodman, MD

Despite the development of many "breakthrough" drugs, heart disease remains the number-one killer of Americans. In *Magnificent Magnesium*, world-renowned cardiologist Dr. Dennis Goodman shines a spotlight on magnesium, the mineral that can maximize your heart health without side effects. The author first establishes a firm foundation for understanding heart disease. Next, he examines the important role magnesium plays in life processes and explores how a deficiency of this substance can lead to many common health conditions. The author then details magnesium's astounding heart-healthy benefits, along with the additional advantages it provides for other diseases. Finally, he offers clear guidelines on how to select and use this mineral to greatest effect.

$14.95 US • 192 pages • 6 x 9-inch paperback • ISBN 978-0-7570-0391-2

Your Blood Never Lies

How to Read a Blood Test for a Longer, Healthier Life

James B. LaValle, RPh, CCN

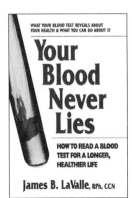

A standard blood test indicates how well the kidneys and liver are functioning, the potential for heart disease, and a host of other vital health markers. Unfortunately, most of us cannot decipher these results ourselves or even formulate the right questions to ask—or we couldn't, until now. *Your Blood Never Lies* clears up the mystery surrounding blood test results. In simple language, Dr. LaValle explains all the information found on these forms, making it understandable and accessible so that you can look at the results yourself and know the significance of each marker.

$16.95 US • 368 pages • 6 x 9-inch paperback • ISBN 978-0-7570-0350-9

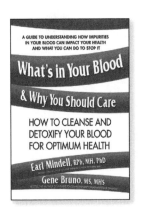

What's In Your Blood & Why You Should Care

How to Cleanse and Detoxify Your Blood for Optimum Health

Earl Mindell, RPh, MH, PhD, and Gene Bruno, Ms, MHS

Like most people, you probably get a blood test and keep your fingers crossed until the results come back. But while these tests focus on key components of your blood, they provide only a limited view of what's going on inside you. Blood tests don't tell you about heavy metals or unwanted pathogens that may be coursing through your body. *What's In Your Blood & Why You Should Care* is the first book to provide a complete picture of the components that make up your blood, how it functions, and what you can do to improve its quality for greater health and longevity. From diets to supplements to medical treatments, it's all there in this groundbreaking book.

$16.95 US • 208 pages • 6 x 9-inch paperback • ISBN 978-0-7570-0443-8